And a Seed was Planted

Volume 3: The context of inclusion
Participatory approaches and research
beyond individual perspectives

And a Seed was Planted

Volume 3: The context of inclusion
Participatory approaches and research
beyond individual perspectives

Edited by
Nick Pollard
Hanneke van Bruggen
Sarah Kantartzis

Forewords by
Sridhar Venkatapuram
and
Elizabeth Townsend

w&b

MMXXIII

© Whiting & Birch Ltd 2023
Published by Whiting & Birch Ltd,
London SE23 3HZ

ISBN 9781861776068 (this volume)
Set ISBN 9781861776242

Contents

Acknowledgements

We would like to thank all the contributors and the people who have worked with them, and with us, to make 'And a seed was planted…' possible. Putting together such a diverse collection of material translated from so many languages and with authors in locations across the world is always challenging, and always worthwhile. Two of our contributors, Linda Wilson and Ellen Ferguson, did not live to see their work published, and we would like to dedicate this project to their memories. There are lots of ways in which we have had help and contributions from our colleagues, friends and families from coffee and a bit of space to work in, to advice, for which we are grateful. We would especially like to thank everyone for persevering with us to publication.

Nick: I would like to thank Linda, Molly, Joshua, Daisy and Olivia for their patience and toleration during this project, including some unusual 'holidays', to facilitate meetings. Thanks also to the Occupational Therapy, Vocational Rehabilitation and Dietetics team and students at Sheffield Hallam University (past and present) for their continued support and interest in this work.

Sarah: Thank you to Christos, Katerina and Harry for your patience and understanding, and to our grandchildren, Lucas and Francesca, that arrived during this project and who give so much love and never ending joy! Thank you also to colleagues at Queen Margaret University Edinburgh for your continual support.

Hanneke: Thank you Sarah and Nick for working together and taking the long road together with all the contributors to the end of this project. Thanks also to Hotze, who patiently listened to me and continued to support me. Thanks to my daughters, Mieke, Floortje and Sanne, who still tolerate that their mother is sometimes "absent" because she "has to" work.

Manifesto for occupation

Hanneke van Bruggen, Nick Pollard, Sarah Kantartzis

Health through occupation

Occupational therapy is about enabling people to do activities that are necessary and important to them and through these to participate in the society of which they are part. 'Occupation' means anything a person *does*. The significance of doing is often overlooked because it is so fundamental to human existence. All our human stories are accounts of things we have done, to become who we are, and the expression of our belonging in a world with others. Through our doing we have constructed, and continue to reconstruct what we do, where, when, how, why and with whom. Occupation, or simply 'doing', is something common to all people everywhere, at all stages of life. It is important not only for what each of us can do in our lifetimes, but also for the kind of world we are building for the future.

There is a fundamental relationship between health and occupation. Through our occupations we are able to orchestrate our lives in ways that enable us not only to survive, but also to develop our potential and express our skills, while creating and maintaining our connections with others. Through our occupation we can develop and maintain our families, neighbourhoods and communities as sources of belonging, opportunities and common action. Occupation therefore is not only important to each individual, but also, through our collective occupation we develop the kind of lives that we live together. Occupation is an essential factor in life quality, and in the experience of being human.

However, occupation does not always lead to such positive and health supporting outcomes, and there are many challenges to meaningful and purposeful occupation for some people. These include disability; illness, trauma and disease; differences in access to food, water, shelter, transport, utilities; relative poverty; differences in social status and citizenship rights; differences in legal status; the economic and social consequences of war and other forms of conflict, climate and climate change; pollution; the planning and development of built structures; the effects of social change arising from shifts in population such as ageing, migration or resulting from disease such as HIV/AIDS; the consequences of disaster; personal tragedy; poor government; economic restructuring. The list is not comprehensive, and the factors can be combined in multiple forms with localised and specific effects.

Our concern is that the link between occupation and health has been consistently overlooked. In occupational therapy there has been an ongoing focus on the impact of illness, disease and trauma on the individual. There has been less attention paid to the social determinants of health and to the impact of social exclusion. Health promoting occupation is a key element in public health and in preventing ill-health. Overlooking this has restricted working with the potential of occupation to express and support human flourishing and develop healthy communities.

We argue that the expression of human health is more than an index of outcomes or therapeutic interventions. We support a view of health as not a stable and normative concept but as unbounded and potentially ever extending, incorporating notions of people's flourishing, the ongoing satisfaction of needs and the development of their potentials as fully included members of the society in which they live. We are calling for a discussion about the value and importance of occupation, not just for occupational therapists alone, but for everyone in health and social care and human sciences. We are calling for a rethink of the way health outcomes relate to personal and collective experiences and human values which are based in the understanding of doing. We need to work with others in reclaiming the value of occupation for all and as an important part of public health.

We are also concerned that the idea of occupation is bigger than can be realised through the profession of occupational therapy. Access to health promoting occupations can be a goal for social changes. These occupations have the potential to be owned by everyone, as they are concerned with how we live together and can be based in shared experiences. However, the knowledge and experience that is common to all is not always valued simply because of its common ownership, so there is a role for some people to critically explore ways to make this value more evident. Again, this should engage both those who are occupational therapists and people who are willing to work with them. The future of evidence for the transformative power of occupation is through co-production, participant action, and the sharing of the discussions about it with others.

A call for change

In order to promote health through occupation we need to work to address the multiple factors that influence people's possibility to engage in health promoting occupation. We need to work together to move forward, to create opportunities for all, to achieve individual and societal flourishing. We need to work in partnership, across sectors, disciplines, political and social divides to create the conditions for change in our education, practice and research. To do this we must:

- Build and maintain active dialogues, and negotiate alliances and strategies with disadvantaged and excluded groups and individuals, disability groups and carers' organisations, practitioners and researchers.
- Effectively campaign for health promoting occupation including participation rights across all levels of disability and social barriers
- Develop different forms of action from protest to social enterprises which exemplify and are underpinned by health-promoting occupation
- Challenge the acceptance of social and the resulting health inequalities, through occupation-based practices and particularly those that incorporate sustainable and inclusive economic growth

Call for contributors

This call for change requires multiple partnerships with many and diverse actions. In considering our own potential contribution to this process we consider that it may be useful to develop a book that will provide both theoretical discussions but also discussion of practical and specific projects and actions. We intend that the book will set out examples of practice, narratives, research and theory which explore, explain and promote the connection between occupation-based practices, social inclusion and health. Our intention is to solicit contributions from a wide range of stakeholders, individuals and chapter-writing teams, including: lay persons, service users, administrators, students, professionals, building a 'tapestry' of experiences and ideas that is not only a textbook but a manual for practice, accessible to all. It will address:

- Understanding the importance of occupation in people's lives and its links with the social determinants of health, public health and prevention.
- Why occupation based practice and occupational therapists? Towards a wider awareness of occupation, and making sense of what occupational therapists might offer community groups.
- How occupation based practice fits in wider perspectives of social inclusion work
- Moving from occupational therapy practice based around individuals to occupation based practice with groups and communities
- The particular characteristics of occupation based practice, including:
- Identifying significant variations with occupational therapy practice in traditional settings, including professional boundaries, compartmentalization of responsibilities and being a community member;
- Recognising change – critical moments and turning points;
- Managing risks and dependency;
- Professionalism and power with vulnerable people as colleagues;
- Managing delegation and responsibility for sustainability;
- Common sense, tacit knowledge and articulating occupation;
- Project and change management, progress and timescales
- Strategies for identifying outcomes for funders, partners and managers;

Thank you

Foreword

The argument that the purpose of politics and the polity is to enable citizens to pursue flourishing lives is most often linked to Aristotle, the ancient Greek philosopher (330 BCE). Centuries of discussions and debates have taken place and still continue regarding various aspects of this argument such as what is a flourishing life, who is included as a citizen, what are the boundaries of politics, what are good processes for governing a polity, and so forth. There has also been much discussion about whether this argument can be reconciled with various religions, including Christianity, as well as the possibility of such an argument in other societal political traditions. For example, tall pillars erected during the reign of the first Buddhist emperor Ashoka (220 BCE) identify various entitlements of citizens and instructions for living a good life.

While it may not be apparent to people outside, academic political philosophy in the Anglo-American world has been thriving over the past few decades because various philosophers have revived the direct conversation with Aristotle and Ashoka by putting forward what they argue to be theories of a good and just society for the modern world. In some cases, individuals have put forward a theory of a just world, or global justice. The person often credited with instigating this activity is John Rawls (1921-2002). In 1971, in his book, *A Theory of Justice*, he laid out critiques of various secular approaches to a good society and then put forward a careful argument for the purpose of some basic social institutions, what citizens are entitled to, how they should engage with each other in mutual cooperation, and so forth.

One of the curious and frustrating things about Rawls's stupendous effort is that he did not give sufficient consideration to health. The state of one's physical and mental functioning directly affects what one can be and do on any given day as well as what plans one can make and the life one can pursue. So how can something so important not be included in the consideration of what public institutions are meant to do, and how fellow members of society should treat each other? One plausible explanation is that Rawls, like many other individuals, particularly in the United States, believed that health is a 'natural good.' Health is seen as something that luck /nature gives to some people or takes away. Health is also something that individuals control through their personal behaviours. And, society addresses poor health through provision of sufficient income to individuals that will allow the purchase of adequate 'healthcare' to return them back to normal functioning. And, without going into much detail, Rawls thought that people who are born severely impaired or who will never return to 'normal' should be dealt with by charitable institutions – not our justice promoting institutions. Given his quite monumental project to articulate a theory of a just and well-ordered society, he was focused on the 'typical' or 'ideal' individual that is able bodied and interested in pursuing a flourishing life. Similarly, he wanted to focus on one society before thinking about a world with many societies, some of which may not even share some of the basic tenets of his just society.

Rawls's theory has received enormous scrutiny resulting in both criticism and praise. Nevertheless, across the discipline and world over, he is credited with bringing back our philosophical attention to the idea of social and global justice, or the question of a good society. Other philosophers have responded to Rawls, and all theories previous to his, by offering their own alternatives. They all start from the point that all human beings are morally equal and value freedom. And from here, different theories focus on what individuals are entitled to from their social environments including public institutions as well as how people should treat each other. Now, while this has been going on in academic literature, it is not hard to see that the same questions are in play in 'real world' politics across the world. Who is included in a society? What are they entitled to? Which institutions are required and which are not? What makes a good institution? How should citizens treat each other?

It is against this background that it is profoundly exciting to see Occupational Science seeking to identify its moral or ethical mission. One could situate Occupational Science as part of health institutions that constitute basic social institutions. That is, Occupational Science is part of a basic social institution whose primary purpose is social justice, or enabling individuals to pursue flourishing lives. Or, more courageously, Occupational Science could aim to stand on its own and assert that it seeks to enable flourishing lives everywhere—within and outside health institutions. Nevertheless, in either case, linking a science to a moral mission requires rigorous and careful reasoning that cuts across the sciences and humanities. And importantly, it requires a clear engagement with a conception or theory of social justice, or a good society. The present volume reflects the kind of deep empirical engagement and mutual reflection between Occupational Science and social justice philosophy we need right now.

I personally feel enormous pride and delight that Occupational Science academics and practitioners have found something helpful in my argument for health justice, and the capabilities approach more generally. While I invite and look forward to further engagement, I also want to encourage a much wider engagement with all the other philosophical approaches to social and global justice. The idea that there is a group of people who believe in and aim to help individuals, particularly those that are marginalized in a society, to be and do things in their lives that they value, should be more widely known and appreciated. Philosophers will benefit from knowing that it is not just a theoretical argument, but embodied in the work of Occupational Science practitioners. And Occupational Science will likely benefit from seeing all the variety of conceptions of justice and how philosophers reason and justify arguments for equity. The present volume represents the start of such an engagement, and I hope, will initiate a new phase in both Occupational Science and in our broader reasoning about social and global justice.

Sridhar Venkatapuram
London

Foreword

What an accomplishment! With *And a Seed was Planted* the European editors and a global array of authors have created a unique book about transforming societies day by day. Here is a book full of ideas and examples for globally minded persons who are committed to engagement 'with' versus doing 'to' others in promoting health, well-being, and justice around the world.

And a Seed was Planted offers a collection of very interesting approaches to complex, global issues based on citizen participation, not relying on top down governmental action. The projects are socially minded with awareness that policies, economics, rituals, and other social structures are at the root of social exclusion, inequity, poverty, and other conditions that persists to this day across parts of Europe, Asia, Africa, South, and North America. It's interesting to consider that some readers may find the approaches described here as ordinary because they are based on engaging people in day-to-day occupations like gardening and employment. Yet these are radical approaches because they challenge the status quo for marginalized or vulnerable groups, like the persons with visual impairments or refugees, whose participation in daily life is restricted beyond their individual conditions. Transformation is of concern here particularly in times and places where disabled people and others face restricted participation, including their lack of voice and choice in health and social services.

This book should attract any practitioner who engages participants in projects with aims for transforming societies anywhere in the world. Hopefully occupational therapists will be especially pleased to see projects that, to me, illustrate the untapped potential of this profession to create an occupationally just world. In seeing occupational therapy's potential with the examples and projects in this book, readers may imagine new ways to link day-by-day life with health, well-being, and daily life.

As an occupational therapist with 50 years experience, I celebrate the book's reclamation of engagement in occupation – action beyond talking – and the commitment to practices that illustrate funding and approaches outside as well as inside medical systems. Despite global job pressures, from salaries and job descriptions to standardized protocols and evidence-based practice based on individualistic, biomedical priorities, the authors present an array of ways in which occupational therapists can break away. Community occupational therapy, government policy-based occupational therapy, justice-oriented occupational therapy, occupational therapy leadership, and related ideas are all championed and legitimized through the authors' stories.

Why am I so enthusiastic? Clearly I love the ideas and practice examples in *And a Seed was Planted*. I also love the accessibility of these in seven clearly organized sections. Section 1 nicely introduces Social Inclusion, Occupation, and Occupation-Based Social Inclusion, plus a story by an artist with a difficult life. The book is more than a collection of practice stories with Section II illuminating *Theoretical Views* related to projects, and Section III on projects that profile *Shifting Perspectives*. Section IV (*Learning Inclusion*) and Section V (*Projects*) together include 12 chapters of wonderful examples of occupation-based social inclusion practices. Beyond the neatness of the book's structure, I also love *Occupation-Based Social Inclusion* because the projects illustrate the intent of the 1948 Declaration of Human Rights (United Nations) with its naming of education, housing, employment, and other everyday sites for doing human rights and justice. Amartya Sen (2009) might see the projects described here as real life ways to reduce what he called 'inclusionary incoherence', referring to gaps between ideas like justice, and everyday realities.

Finally, congratulations are due to the team that made *Occupation-Based Social Inclusion* possible. After what must have been many hours of collaboration, translation, and editing, the editors and authors can be proud of their invaluable gift to the English-reading world. With their efforts, English-readers are privileged to learn about innovative approaches to occupation-based social inclusion around the world.

Elizabeth Townsend, PhD, OTRegPEI, FCAOT
Professor Emerita, Dalhousie University
Liz.Townsend@Dal.ca
Adjunct Professor, University of Prince Edward Island
etownsend@upei.ca

Prologue to Volume 3
The Context of Inclusion:
Participatory approaches and research beyond individual perspectives

Occupational therapy originated in social reform, but early in its history became allied with medicine, a biomedical perspective and a focus on individual health. Over the last two decades the profession has recognised the value of the work of its pioneers and argued for principles such as occupational justice and the right to health-promoting occupations, social inclusion, and for forms of involvement based in the community which centre around people doing things together for social change. In *'And a seed was planted...' Occupation based approaches for social inclusion* the Editors have set out to show how these ideas are being put into practice internationally.

This is the final volume of a three-volume set. The first volume opened with three chapters in which the Editors offer an introduction to the main concepts discussed throughout the set – social inclusion, occupation, and approaches to occupation-based social inclusion. A further two sections offered chapters on Theoretical Views and Shifting Perspectives.

The second volume took these ideas in two sections, Learning Inclusion, exploring occupation-based learning experiences in diverse settings, and Projects presenting accounts of community-based projects in different stages of development.

This is the third volume of this three-volume set. It is organised in two sections. Contributors in the first section, The Context of Inclusion, discuss the multiple determinants influencing possibilities for inclusion, including policy, historico-cultural and economic influences, as well as institutional structures, with chapters located in Africa, Asia, Europe and North America. A final section discusses examples of participatory approaches, exploring innovative ways of knowing, including storytelling and design, as well as participatory processes and the doing of research as an occupation.

About the authors

Rocco Angarola, BSc (Hons), MSc, Occupational Therapist, NHS Lothian, Scotland.

Ricky Buchanan, Disabled Person, assistive technology blogger, and noncompliant research participant.

Marijke Burger, MSc Orthopedagogy & behavioral studies, member of "Family Council (mental healthcare)GGZ InGeest", Service User, The Netherlands.

Barbara Casparie, BSc., Service User, Zuyd University of Applied Sciences, The Netherlands.

Paul Chamberlain, Professor of Design, Co-Director C3RI, Head of Art and Design Research Centre, Director of Lab4Living and Director of Design Futures, Sheffield Hallam University, UK

Claire Craig, Professor of Design and Creative Practice and Co-Director, Lab4Living, Sheffield Hallam University, UK.

Emma Crawford, PhD, Lecturer in Occupational Therapy, School of Health and Rehabilitation Sciences, Faculty of Health and Behavioural Sciences, University of Queensland, Australia.

Maarten de Wit, PhD., Service User/ Researcher, Stichting TOOLS, VU Medical Centre, Amsterdam, The Netherlands.

Krishna Gautam, Secretary General of CIL (Independent Living Centre) Kathmandu, Nepal

Jyothi Gupta, PhD, OTR/L, FAOTA, Chair and Professor, Department of Occupational Therapy, School of Health Professions, University of Texas Medical Branch, Galveston, TX, USA.

Anthony Isaac, Indigenous Services Manager, Student Services Department, Okanagan College, British Columbia, Canada.

Michael Kenko Iwama, PhD OT(C), Professor / Chief Program Strategist, Occupational Therapy Doctorate Division, School of Medicine, Duke University, USA.

Chikako Koyama, PhD, Professor of Occupational Therapy, Prefectural University of Hiroshima, Japan.

Debbie Laliberte Rudman, Distinguished University Professor, School of Occupational Therapy & Graduate Program in Health and Rehabilitation Sciences (Occupational Science field), University of Western Ontario, Canada.

Natasha Layton, PhD, Occupational therapist, Senior Research Fellow with the Rehabilitation, Ageing and Independent Living (RAIL) Research Centre, Monash University, Australia.

Amy Lynch, PhD, OTR/L, Program Coordinator, International Adoption Health Program at the Children's Hospital of Philadelphia. Assistant Professor, Occupational Therapy, Temple University, USA

Fambaineni Innocent Magweva, former Executive director of the National Association of Societies for the Care of the Handicapped, Harare, Zimbabwe, passed away during the preparation of this book.

Tatenda John Maphosa, Senior Rehabilitation Consultant, Procare Group, Deakin, Australia Capital Territory.

Alexandra McCallum, PhD Candidate at Griffith University, Australia.

Tecla Mlambo, PhD, Lecturer in Occupational Therapy University of Zimbabwe College of Health Sciences, Harare, Zimbabwe.

Albine Moser, PhD, MPH, RN, Senior Researcher, Zuyd University of Applied Sciences, The Netherlands.

Nyaradzai Munambah, PhD, University of Zimbabwe Faculty of Medicine and Health Sciences, Rehabilitation Sciences Unit, Harare, Zimbabwe.

Rhona Murray, Retired Social Care Managing Director, Scotland.

Clement Nhunzvi, PhD, University of Zimbabwe Faculty Medicine and Health Sciences, Rehabilitation Sciences Unit, Harare, Zimbabwe.

Treena Orchard, Associate Professor & Undergraduate Chair School of Health Studies, University of Western Ontario, Canada.

Alvin Ng Lai Oon, PhD, Associate Dean (International) School of Medical and Life Sciences and Professor, Department of Psychology, Sunway University, Malaysia.

Jennifer S. Pitonyak, PhD, OTR/L, SCFES, Director and Associate Professor, School of Occupational Therapy, Pacific University, Oregon, USA

Barbara Piškur, PhD, MSc. OT., Senior Researcher, Zuyd University of Applied Sciences, The Netherlands.

Esther Stoffers, MSc, Service User Representative, MET GGZ, The Netherlands.

Chantelle Richmond, Associate Professor, Department of Geography, University of Western Ontario, Canada.

Debra Rybski, PhD, MSHCA, OTR/L, Associate Professor and Chair Department of Occupational Science & Occupational Therapy, Doisy College of Health Sciences, Saint Louis University, USA

Steven D. Taff, PhD., OTR/L. Associate Director of Professional Education and Academic Affairs. Assistant Professor in Occupational Therapy & Medicine, Washington University School of Medicine, USA

Masayuki Takagi, PhD, Associate Professor of Occupational Therapy, Prefectural University of Hiroshima, Japan.

Erin Wilson, PhD, Professor and Uniting Chair in Community Services Innovation at the Centre for Social Impact Swinburne. School of Business, Law and Entrepreneurship, Swinburne University of Technology, Australia.

Teoh Jou Yin, MRCOT, FHEA, Senior Lecturer, Occupational Therapy Division, Brunel University London.

Hiromi Yoshikawa, PhD, Professor of Occupational Therapy, Prefectural University of Hiroshima, Japan.

Tsutako Yoshikawa is an older Japanese woman.

Section 6
The context of inclusion: Working beyond individual perspectives

This section includes discussion of the multiple determinants influencing possibilities for inclusion, including policy and changes in policy, historico-cultural influences, socio-economic structures and institutional structures. With chapters from Japan, Zimbabwe, Nepal, Malaysia, USA and Scotland, UK, this section provides a rich insight into the diversity but also the commonalities as people work to promote inclusive opportunities and provide a critical lens on the structures in which these are occurring.

This section opens with the story of Hiromi Yoshikawa and her mother as, situated within the cultural context of Japan, they navigate their way through the services available to the elderly in striving to maintain a life that is seen to be meaningful and relevant.

In the following chapter Gupta et al. discuss the multiple social and environmental factors in childhood that can negatively impact on development, creating conditions of injustice and exclusion in the United States. They conceptualise health as comprising of multiple determinants and urge occupational therapists to work with these multiple determinants in order to facilitate optimal development and inclusion for all children. They indicate the role played by current reimbursement practices of the health care industry in restricting occupational therapy practice to health care settings at the expense of practice that will address some of the wider determinants of children's development.

Next Teoh et al. reflects on the impact of culture on the possibilities for inclusion for blind and visually impaired people in conservative Malaysian Chinese families. Their discussion illuminates the complexity of the intertwinings of historical, economic and social factors in the development of beliefs, values and customs together with the individual and specific ways that these are enacted in daily life.

Whereas Teoh et al. focus on the family, the following chapter by Murray focuses on the institutional frameworks that have structured the opportunities for inclusion of people with learning disabilities in the UK, and specifically in Scotland. Taking a historical perspective Murray traces the changing approaches to care, from institutional to community based living, but warns that despite increased opportunities currently for autonomy and engagement in the occupation in the community, such services remain at risk of economic and political change.

Mlambo et al. provide a detailed discussion of the legislative and policy framework supporting occupation-based social inclusion in Zimbabwe while recognising the potential gap between policy and implementation. They recognise the importance of legislation that not only provides guidance but that also demands implementation, as

---

well as the significance of an organised structure of groups representing persons with disability (from the local to the national) that can advocate for change. In reflecting on contemporary occupational therapy in Zimbabwe they highlight the contextual issues that have influenced the traditional focus of practice on acute medical settings, while indicating some of the ways that they are working to expand beyond this to address some of the broader social and health issues affecting the population.

The final chapter in this section comes from Nepal and outlines the activities of the Independent Living Organisation (CIL-Kathmandu). This chapter demonstrates the determination of the members of the organisation to work for their rights to independent living in their own communities, to services that are supportive of their needs, and their active work to tackle not only architectural barriers, but also attitudinal, communication and institutional barriers. The chapter also demonstrates the fragility of such efforts at times of crisis, such as the natural disaster of the earthquake of 2015.

Chapter 1
Aging with disabilities in Japan:
How to overcome isolation and boredom

Hiromi Yoshikawa, Chikako Koyama,
Masayuki Takagi, and Tsutako Yoshikawa

I, Hiromi, am the first author. I am an occupational therapist and a university professor. Koyama, the second author, has worked with me for 20 years. She is seven years younger than me. Takagi, the third author, was my student. We work at the same university. This is the story of my mother, Tsutako. My involvement with her is both as a daughter and as an occupational therapist. Koyama's involvement is as a friend of her daughter. Takagi's involvement with her is through her participation in an inclusive community group he has established.

Life after developing disabilities

My mother is an old Japanese woman with disabilities. She had a traffic accident at the age of 66 in 1997. She had surgery for her fractures of both legs and received noninvasive treatment for a fracture of the pelvis. After four months she was discharged from a hospital, but needed a walking frame to walk. She has since taken several falls, with two fractures of the distal end of the radius, the ischium, and compression fractures of the lumbar. After some of these falls she was bedridden for a while.

The Long-Term Care Insurance Act for older people with disabilities was established in 2000 (Ministry of Health, Labour and Welfare, 2002), although the act is primarily for family care givers rather than people with disabilities. It includes services such as care facilities, nursing homes, day care, and visiting care. There are two categories in the functional level of clients: those who need support and those who need care. Support-needs are determined as either level 1 or 2, whereas care-needs levels range between 1 and 5. Level 1 means the mildest disabilities and level 5 means the severest disabilities.

The Long-Term Care Insurance Act established a training programme for care managers. Social workers, nurses, and therapists become care managers through completion of this programme under the Act. The care manager plans how often and what kinds of services a client uses based on assessments. The maximum costs for each level are decided by law. Service users pay ten percent of the total cost. An aim of this act was to convey the idea that caring for older people with disabilities should be a social issue rather than a family issue. Traditionally, the eldest son takes responsibilities for caring for his parents, but actually his wife would care for them. Currently unmarried children often care for their parents. Care giving by family members is unpaid work, and caregivers can't earn enough money to live on. Because of the rising care cost at a time of economic stringency combined with an especially steep rise in the average age of the Japanese population, the government is afraid of increased social security expenses (Ministry of Health, Labour and Welfare, 2015).

My mother's care-needs were assessed at level 2 at first. She has had to have her level certified every six months or annually. The level is reassessed annually for every person registered in the Act. Most older people with disabilities just stay around their bed and their level is at first stable and then gets worse. My mother's level has changed often, because she is more active. Sometimes she is more independent but becomes more dependent after taking a fall. Her care-needs level has been at level 1 and her support-needs at level 2 most of the time. She went to a day care center twice a week for nearly ten years. There she made craft items, played games and sang songs. Although those activities did not appeal to her, she liked talking with people. She had several friends there, but she lost them because their conditions were getting worse. All the people in the day care center had complex illnesses combined with other disabilities or conditions, such as dementia, Parkinson's disease, and cerebral infarction. She tried to understand when a person said illogical things. For example, one friend had a grandchild who was an elementary school student and might visit her home, yet another day he became a university student. I explained that her friend probably had dementia. She said that she might have mild dementia, but she was a very nice person. My mother helped her to open her bag of medication and take off her clothes. I knew about the progress of her disease when my mother talked about her. This friend was one of those who had ceased to come to the day care center.

Several times my mother traveled with me by train. Her physical therapists had trained her in climbing stairs during individual rehabilitation sessions in the day care center, so she could manage stairs in train stations. She recognized that stair training was more useful for her getting around than range of motion exercises, but she didn't say this because she supposed that her physical therapist preferred therapeutic approaches. She thought that stair training is too ordinary to be provided by her physical therapist with a national licensure. When her level of support needs was assessed as lower, her individual session was shortened. My mother continued to receive range of motion exercises but stair training stopped. She was upset but said nothing.

One day she became wet when going to the toilet. The day care center staff gave her clothes to change into. Although the toilet was broken, day care center group members thought that she had been incontinent. They laughed. My mother tried to explain what had happened. They said laughingly that they knew, she didn't have to explain. She has never gone there since then. She doesn't want to belong to the group.

She took a fall again. She had to adapt to a life in bed again. I didn't bring her to a hospital based on my clinical reasoning. I decided through interview, observation, and manual examination that a medical doctor's diagnosis was not needed. Two months later when she could move, I brought her to a hospital. An orthopaedist diagnosed a compression fracture of the lumbar vertebrae. She received physical therapy services once a week for two months. Then her physical therapist recommended that she use a day care center. Reducing medical costs is another reason for establishing the Long-Care Term Insurance Act. The government tried to transfer rehabilitation services for older people with disabilities from the medical insurance to care insurance earlier

(Ministry of Health, Labour and Health, 2009). My mother's care needs were certified at level 4. She went to another day care center. She had individual rehabilitation sessions from both physical and occupational therapists. Both therapists did the same exercises such as standing up and sitting down and muscle stretching.

When she was reassessed a year later her support-needs were certified at level 1. According to changes in the Long-Term Care Insurance Act made by the national government in April 2015, local governments now have to decide whether they pay for services for persons in support-needs or establish a new programme for them. My local government has not decided how to adopt these changes. Consequently, the day care center no longer provides services which are not covered by the government either at national or local level. Even though she was thinking of leaving the new center my mother felt bad when it refused to give her any more services.

Now she is doing laundry, cleaning rooms, some cooking, caring for a cat, watering plants, reading books and newspapers, and watching television, after she quit the day care center. She is independent at home, but she can't walk outside of her house because of fatigue and fear of cars in the road. She doesn't talk because most days there are no visitors.

A caregiver as a daughter and an occupational therapist

I am an only child. My father left after financial problems when I was 16 years old. My mother raised me until I began working as an occupational therapist. We had lived separately for more than 15 years. She moved from Nagano to Hiroshima, 700 kilometers west from her hometown when I became a teacher at my current university in 1995. My mother and I started living together because she said she was tired of living alone after retirement. She had enjoyed travelling to her hometown after moving to my place until the accident. After the accident I became a caregiver. Although I thought I knew a lot of things about the theory of care and rehabilitation after fracture, I encountered the real situation and learned new knowledge from this experience.

One day, I found her smiling when I visited her at the hospital. She told me that she had been to a toilet using a wheelchair by herself. I felt angry and cried because I knew that at her level of independence she needed moderate assistance for transfers and toileting. I also knew that many patients at the same level as her experienced falls. I told her about the risk of falling and insisted that she never did it again. She became angry and said 'I'm not stupid. I only do what I can do.' I realized that through concerns with risk managements therapists had taken the opportunities from people with disabilities to have control over what they want to do.

After her discharge from the hospital, she did household tasks using a walking frame. She invented new ways to do them, such as reorganizing the steps of the process and using new equipments such as a sock aid and a reacher. She transported her laundry from the washing machine for drying with a walking frame, which she used like a cart. Around ten months after her discharge, she said that her walking frame had become heavy. Then she couldn't pick it up. I realized later the reason was that her center of gravity had moved forward because of the restriction on her range of hip motion. She used lordosis of the lumbar to compensate for the hip restriction so that she had severe pain in her lumbar region. She became bedridden. I stayed home from work.

I thought about the best way for my mother and me to live together. I asked her to change a diaper by herself on the bed. My mother and I practiced so that she could independently manage excretion while in bed. Then she could also use a urinal by herself. Thus I kept working while she was bedridden.

Staying in bed for a month cured the hip restriction and pain without diagnosis and physical therapy. We have overcome these troubles several times when she became bedridden because of pain. My perspective of my mother taking a fall has been changed from failing to prevent them to managing an event which often occurs in her life. When I heard from my mother or somebody else that she had fallen, at first I imagined the worst situation, then several options that I could put into effect. Imagining the worst scenario at first is my strategy for being ready to accept the situation.

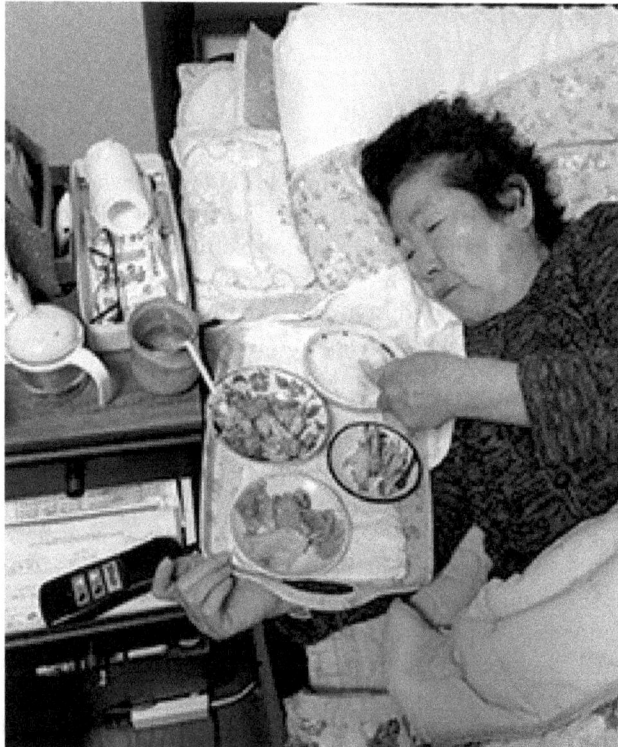

Photo 1 : Eating in the bed

I feel still some guilt when I have to be away from home, especially if it is more than a week. I asked professional carers to look after my mother. The expense of these services is covered by the Long-Term Care Insurance Act. She accepted their assistance while she was bedridden. I hired professional carers again when she was independent in her personal care because she couldn't go shopping for groceries. I also wanted them to watch out for her. She complained that they didn't do anything and just charged her. I explained that I asked them because I worry about her. I want to know whether she is safe or not. She said, 'It's your issue. Be prepared.' I imagined the end of her life and myself at her funeral.

Social environments

Boredom is another problem for my mother. She likes talking to people and having social exchanges, but there is nobody at home. She made some personal rapport with some of the professional carers with whom she could talk about her interests and share things about families and hobbies. Although keeping private considerations out of the professional life is recommended in the educational programme of health care service providers, establishing a personal rapport with my mother is essential for the therapist who intends to work with her. She wants to meet a person, not merely a depersonalized professional.

Koyama maintains a good relationship with my mother. When my mother was transferred to a hospital after the accident, Koyama went to the hospital because I was out of the city. She always helped me. My mother calls Koyama on the phone when I am out of the office and she is looking for me. She sometimes visits and stays with my mother during my absence. My mother likes to talk to her. My mother checks the daily fortune telling column in the newspaper every day about Koyama, me, and herself.

Koyama has experiences of caring for her grandmother. The end of her grandmother's life at a hospital after she took a fall was regrettable. She deteriorated and became unconscious over several weeks, and passed away. Koyama often visited my mother because of the unease over the death of her grandmother.

Koyama talks about my mother. 'I enjoy hearing her stories. When she talks she talks humorously about the people in the day care center and her neighbours. Sometimes she says this is secret from her daughter.'

I thank Koyama but I am afraid of pressing her to care for my mother because my position at work is higher than hers. I asked other people such as a neighbour and a graduate student[1] to visit my mother during my absence. I will continue to try to ask different people. I still want someone to watch out for her. I want her to get along with the persons I ask to visit her. She said that being alone is better than staying with a person who she doesn't like.

My mother has hearing difficulties with aging and after otitis media, and wears a hearing aid. People should practice talking to people wearing hearing aids. A person wearing a hearing aid can only hear voices one meter away. Most people don't know that it is important to make the context of communication clear for effective understanding. They talk loudly and make sounds one by one. My mother doesn't recognize what they are saying. As a result, there are a lot of misunderstandings.

Creating opportunities for occupations

Takagi manages a programme making crafts named Mono-Zukuri Kobo Sakura twice a month for community citizens. *Mono* means things and *zukuri* means making. *Kobo* is a space like a workshop in which things are made by people. *Saku* means making and *ra* means people. *Sakura* shares its pronunciation with the Japanese word for cherry blossom. Cherry blossom is the cultural symbol for the beginning of something and a gathering of people in the spring which we call 'Hana-Mi'. I bring my mother to the programme. Most of the participants of the programme are healthy older people. She makes rattan work which she had learned to do in her 50s. She enjoys talking with people. If someone admires her work when she finishes, she gives it to them. She teaches some of them how to make rattan work. She brings pickles she has made for other participants. Positive feelings and social exchanges contribute to her emotional and social well-being.

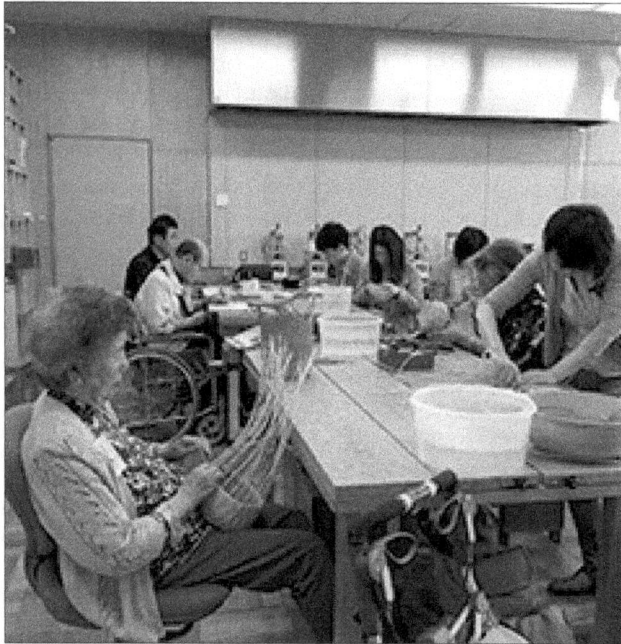

Photo 2: Making a basket at Mono-Zukuri Kobo Sakura

Takagi has been interested in non-traditional practice areas of occupational therapy since he was a student. He established computer classes for residents of a long-term care facility who had severe disabilities. The lives of those persons in an institution are restricted both physically and socially. At the beginning of the computer class the residents couldn't wait for the screen to brighten after turning it on. They tried to move the cursor on the screen with their hands instead of using a mouse. Pad style daily calendars were produced at the end of class three months later. Every person wrote something and put illustrations or photos on each date in the calendar. The residents were assessed using the Canadian Occupational Performance Measure, the Goal Attainment Scale, and health-related quality of life measured by the SF-36 (Takagi, 2008) and produced increased scores after the activity. Participants could write letters to their family and keep journals using a computer. Participation in the computer class changed their life styles. One person quit smoking because he wanted to buy his own computer. The perspectives of staff in the facility toward those residents changed from seeing them as receivers of care to becoming makers of something. The staff acquired computers and rearranged the computer area.

Wicks (2008) introduced how occupational perspectives spread in the community. Takagi studied in the Australasian Occupational Science Center for years after his research in the long term care facility where he was supervised by Alison Wicks. He participated in a Men's Shed and made wood work products in Australia. He realized that inclusive occupational opportunities are needed in a community.

After his study in Australia Takagi organized a programme for citizens called 'Things I Can Do for Myself and Society for Citizens'. This was sponsored by the Prefectural University of Hiroshima. After a year the citizens who attended the programme established a group named Go for Mihara. Mihara is the name of our city. The group became core members in the organizing of Mono-Zukuri Kobo Sakura. The programme participants are diverse in age, sex, and disability. Outpatients of the university clinic were also referred to attend. They include retired people, housewives, persons with disabilities such as hemiplegia and Parkinson's disease and my mother. The policies of the programme are that participants select what they make, teach each other, and bring materials. Participants use the facilities and tools in the university. There are many kinds of activities such as making bags of paper or cloth, sewing, painting, origami, pottery and woodworking. Some products from the programme were sold in the university festival[2]. Students in the occupational therapy department of the university participate in the programme as a part of their course work for almost a year.

Takagi talked about my mother. 'Your mother makes the group more inclusive. People care about your mother and she cares about them. My vision is to establish an inclusive community. I want to make groups that anybody can participate in regardless of whether they are old or young and have a disability or not.'

Conclusion

I can help my mother, as an occupational therapist and as her daughter, in enabling occupations such as self-care and household activities. Doing these occupations might be restricted through practices of risk management and precautionary measures from a professional point of view.

My mother, Tsutako said. 'I'm going to be 85 years old. It's difficult to have an idea what I want to do because of disabilities and cold weather. I want to find something while I'm waiting for spring. I always think that something I can do will be the one to live for. I expect that my daughter will take me to some places for watching cherry blossom at Hana-Mi. I think about memories of my hometown because I live far away from there. The memories are important but I want to enjoy my life here. I can find some friends and talk them through Mono-Zukuri. It is the most enjoyable.'

She has lost her freedom to get around and do things with her friends as she gets older. Koyama contributes through maintaining a person to person relationship. Takagi contributes by establishing a new social environment in the community. Both are necessary for isolated people like my mother. She had lost friends even when she lived in her hometown through the process of getting old. It is difficult to find new relationships. Inclusive community programmes will support isolated people. The other people who join the programme know that each person can do something regardless of their age and disabilities. It is important to have opportunities for sharing their experiences. The knowledge and skills of occupational therapists can contribute to social inclusion by helping people to do what they want to do and establishing and organizing occupational opportunities for diverse people.

Notes

1   Building a social network is not easy in Japan. Neighbours may help each other if they have lived in the same community for a long time. I can only ask a few neighbours to look after my mother during my absence. She was a nurse and moved from the east of Japan. I have sometimes invited some graduate students who have the time and live nearby to my house. The students ate dishes which my mother cooked.
2   Japanese universities usually have a festival once a year organized by students. There are shops of crafts and food, concert, and comedy events. Neighbours and parents of students visit universities at the festival.

References

Ministry of Health, Labour and Welfare (2002) *Long-term Care Insurance in Japan.* [Accessed 20 September 2015 at http://www.mhlw.go.jp/english/topics/elderly/care]

Ministry of Health, Labour and Welfare (2015) *Health and Medical Services in Annual Health, Labour and Welfare Report 2013-2014* [Accessed 30 January, 2016 at http://www.mhlw.go.jp/english/wp/wp-hw8/]

Ministry of Health, Labour and Welfare (2009) *Establishing a Stable Sustainable Health Insurance System in Annual Health, Labour and Welfare Report 2007-2008* [Accessed 30 January, 2016 at http://www.mhlw.go.jp/english/wp/wp-hw2/index.html]

Takagi, T. and Yoshikawa, H. (2008) A computer-based programme for residents of facilities for persons with physical disabilities: The effects on occupational performance and feelings of health. *The Journal of Japanese Occupational Therapy Association,* 27, 5, 522-532

Wicks, A. (2008) Into the main stream: Making occupational science visible. *The Japanese Journal of Occupational Science,* 2, 7-17 [Accessed 20 September, 2015 at http://www.jsso.jp/JJOS/JJOS2(1)/JJOS2(1)-04.pdf]

Chapter 2
Enhancing occupational potential and health: A life-course health development approach

Jyothi Gupta, Amy Lynch, Jennifer Pitonyak, Debra Rybski and Steven D. Taff

Introduction

Early adversity in childhood is characterized by exposure to multiple, complex risk factors, such as neglect, abuse, poverty, and racial discrimination, that transact with policies to create an environment of toxic stress. The Life Course Health Development (LCHD) model (Halfon & Hochstein, 2002; Halfon & Forrest, 2018.) is a useful framework for explaining the impact of early exposure to adverse life situations and toxic stress, their relationship with critical periods of development that negatively impacts the health development trajectory, and puts the individual at risk of occupational injustice and social exclusion. The LCHD model conceptualizes health as an outcome of multiple determinants nested in transacting family, community, and policy contexts, what Halfon and Hochstein (2002) term a nested environment. While exposure to a single risk factor may not significantly alter health development, when multiple risks transact individuals face adversity that excludes participation in desired, health-producing occupations. We apply the LCHD model to illustrate how multiple, compounded risks in early childhood enhances the likelihood of occupational injustices and social exclusion throughout the life course.

The term *toxic stress* indicates early, significant and sustained stress on the developing child through recurrent traumatic events such as abuse, violence, homelessness, unsafe neighborhoods or chronic poverty (Shonkoff, 2012). Toxic stress has been identified as a key overarching factor in creating early adversity for children, youth and families that negatively impact their ability to experience social inclusion. Toxic stress environments and adverse experiences literally alter brain architecture in early childhood resulting in long-term physiological, cognitive and psychological damage (Shonkoff, 2012). The environments that cultivate toxic stress are also those that tend to result in patterns of social exclusion and occupational injustice. Early adverse experiences and consequences of toxic stress are truly lifespan issues that can negatively impact participation in meaningful occupations (Gronski et al, 2013). Childhood toxic stress is an emerging area of practice for occupational therapists, which requires focus on family and broader community support systems to facilitate social inclusion and integration. While the specific stressors may vary according to culture, geography, policy and sociopolitical climate, the complexity of toxic stress makes it essential that it be viewed as a public health issue that crosses ethnic, national, and professional boundaries.

Social exclusion can lead to occupational injustice and negative health trajectories, widening of disparities and ingraining harmful patterns on physical, emotional, and social well-being. Occupational potential develops over time, is influenced by environmental factors, and is dependent upon occupational participation (Wicks, 2005; Pitonyak et al, 2020; Pitonyak et al 2021). Early adversity, therefore, drastically limits occupational potential at the start of the lifespan and during critical periods of development; this pattern sets in motion a less than optimal trajectory. In this chapter, the authors suggest the suitability of the multifactorial LCDH model (Halfon et al, 2014; Halfon & Hochstein, 2002), as a conceptual lens to tackling early adversity to enhance the occupational potential of children, youth, and their families. When the LCHD model is applied to occupational potential, participation in meaningful occupations is itself a therapeutic health determinant. The LCDH model offers a framework through which barriers and facilitators to occupational potential can be examined in relationship to health and social inclusion. The exemplars in this chapter are each identified risk factors for overall poorer occupational and health outcomes-- lack of family permanency through foster care and institutionalization, family homelessness, racial segregation, and inability to engage in early family bonding occupational experiences. The transaction of early risk factors creates a nested environment of toxic stress and social exclusion from achievement of occupational potential across the lifespan.

Delayed permanency:
Impacts of foster care, institutional care, and multiple living transitions

Children removed from their biological homes or placed by biological caregivers into institutional systems experience numerous early adversities that negatively impact development of brain, behavior, and physical, and social well-being. This section discusses three examples of adversities experienced by this group. First, children living in dysfunctional environments may experience adversity in the form of inconsistency of caregiver presence, victims or witnesses to violence, physical or emotional abuse, and neglect. These factors prevent children from developing key neurons for attachment, self-regulation, and development (Drury et al, 2012). Second, these children experience limited access to regular healthcare and quality nutrition (Forkey & Szilagyi, 2014; Mekonnen et al, 2009). Third, the actual transitions between multiple living environments until establishment of a permanent home pose yet another adversity. Risks associated with the social injustices experienced by these children restrict successful and satisfactory participation in individual and family based occupations across their lifespan (Forkey & Szilagyi, 2014; Paul-Ward, 2009).

Risks of early adversity in light of social and occupational injustices call for a keen understanding by interventionists serving these children. Adverse environments experienced by the child in foster care, institutional living, and multiple living situations impact a child's social and emotional development leading to behavioral issues that stem from low self-worth, impaired attachment, poor communication and social engagement skills (Anda, et al, 2006). These behavioral problems greatly limit positive interactions and co-occupations with new parents, siblings, teachers, and peers. The sensory and caregiving deprivation of early adversity impacts the development of the central nervous system (Beckes et al, 2015), and in turn the physical health, sensory integrity, and overall attention and self-regulation. The summative effect of emotional and material deprivation constrains a child from developing the prerequisite skills to participate in daily occupations such as dressing, home and school play, and community sporting. Additionally, early adversity threatens the learning and establishment of solid foundational skills for information processing and cognitive development. These characteristics reduce a child's potential to succeed in academic environments (Jee et al, 2008) and vocational settings (Pecora et al, 2006). In the context of health development, children who have experienced early adversity have experienced deprivation in physical, social, family, cultural and policy environments.

Global, national and state specific policies that disrupt biological parental rights as well as policies that govern foster care systems, slow a child's access to a stable, permanent home (O'Reilly et al, 2005). Unfortunately, this means that children experience longer periods of non-family living or dysfunctional family living situations before adoption into a stable household. At a family level, the adoption of a child who has experienced early adversity sets in motion a late onset model of shared family occupations. This delay in the establishment and integrity of occupations for both parent and child may impact child and family bonding which in turn can propel early adversity risks to a greater societal issue (Taussig et al, 2012; Paul-Ward, 2009). At a societal level, early adversity impacts establishment of an individual's ability to adequately fulfill their social roles and responsibilities. They are at risk for low levels of education that puts them at risk for earnings below poverty levels, employment that does not include health insurance benefits, and homelessness (Pecora et al, 2006).

It is vital that occupational therapists supporting children who experienced early adversity understand the long-term consequences of early childhood deprivation on the social, psychological, physical health and well being of the child into adulthood. Occupational therapy practice largely is focused on the individual. The LCHD model provides a rationale for establishing macro and micro context stability for therapists working in 'at risk for disruption' homes as well as for the new parent and the child entering a permanent home (Halfon et al, 1992). Occupational therapists can advocate for changes to policy regarding adoption and fostering processes for earlier permanency plans, and appropriate services for children and families.

Family homelessness

In 2013, the US reported 2.5 million children as homeless, an alarming 8% increase over the 2012 census count, representing one out of every 30 children (Bassuk et al, 2014). Children who are homeless are more often hungry, sick, and likely to live with a single mother, who has experienced mental health problems, abuse or sustained trauma (Bassuk et al, 2014). Up to 26% of preschool children and 40% of school age homeless children exhibited mental health problems (Bassuk et al, 2015). Many preschool children who experience homelessness show delays in foundational skills of executive function and self-regulation (Herbers et al, 2014) impairing health and developmental trajectories (Halfon et al, 2014). These adversities can decrease participation and social inclusion, further creating obstacles for health and learning (Whiteford & Pereira, 2012).

Children who are homeless experience disruptions in daily occupations, routines and habits such as eating and hygiene, going to school and spending time with family and friends which can interrupt health development trajectories (Halfon et al, 2014). They experience a loss of collective family support as a result of common shelter rules that require parents to be married and boys older than sixteen to move out. Social disruption of family relationships and supports results in diminished connectedness (Townsend & McWhirter, 2005; Whiteford & Pereira, 2012). Furthermore, a single parent in a shelter must focus on securing financial resources to return to permanent housing. Efforts to obtain and retain work, in particular for women on welfare and in low skilled jobs, creates long periods of time away from children, disrupting and diminishing responsive care giving, essential for optimal child health, development and academic achievement.

Supporting families in shelter programs using a LCHD framework (Halfon et al, 2014) ideally builds on the inherent strengths of the family (Moodie & Ramos, 2014) to facilitate child health and development. Caring relationships provided by not only mothers, but also extended kin, and community caregivers can provide protective supports. Care giving is protective when it is responsive, sensitive and positive (National Scientific Council on the Developing Child [NSCDC], 2015). Protective care giving can be further enhanced by the two generation approach of family support (Lombardi et al, 2014). Supporting parents in turn enhances child development. When parental access to education, economic and social capital increases, children's stress is reduced and healthy development is enhanced (NSCDC, 2010). The two-generation approach builds a young child's social inclusion, through parental support of their child's increased engagement in daily occupations such as self care, emergent literacy, family chores, social skills, and play. This, in turn builds children's capacities for self-regulation (Herbers et al, 2014), and executive function (Diamond & Lee, 2011), essential constructs necessary for successful future social and school inclusion (Cutuli & Herbers, 2014).

In families who experience homelessness, occupational therapists can promote parent-child connectedness and social inclusion (Townsend & McWhirter, 2005) by enhancing bonds with family and community. Care giving training to mothers who are homeless provided by occupational therapists with an understanding of bio-behavioral adaptations (Halfon et al, 2014) to adverse experiences can enhance a mother's capacity to engage in personal and family health promotion (Hopper et al, 2010). Learning to value, recognize personal strengths and care for self, in turn facilitates capability (Alexander, 2008), a social inclusion capacity that can build responsive care giving skills.

Responsive care, in turn, supports child resilience, diminishes risks and fosters healthy development in young children who are homeless (NSCDC, 2015). Yet some children in the face of toxic stress (NSCDC, 2005) need enhanced support to reach optimal participation and social inclusion. Early intervention programs identify developmental delays in children and provide subsequent intervention to enhance child health and development trajectories. Yet only 10% of eligible children received early intervention services (Rosenberg et al, 2008). Further outreach to enhance early identification of young children at risk for social exclusion due to the combined challenges of disability and homelessness can be offered to families in community screenings and private and Federal community programs (Rybski & Wilder, 2008).

The McKinney Vento Homeless Children's Act (2002, 2010), a federal law, requires school districts to identify and provide services to children who are homeless or highly mobile. Occupational therapists can explore roles within horizontally integrated health and education services (Halfon et al, 2014), in early detection of learning issues and help children who experience homelessness develop resilient capacities. Helping families cultivate daily health/school routines and positive, meaningful activities in and after school can support a child's social inclusion in school (Cutuli & Herbers, 2014) which sets up a positive trajectory for economic participation and social inclusion across the lifespan (Whiteford & Pereira 2012; Duncan et al, 2010).

Residential segregation and racism

Poverty is a significant risk factor for poor health and in the United States persons of color are disproportionately poor and bear the burden of mortality and morbidity (Centers for Disease Control and Prevention, 2013). Despite civil rights legislation in the 1960s, many African Americans today contend with segregated neighborhoods, racial discrimination, income inequality, unstable housing, under-resourced schools, inadequate access to health and social services that manifest as health inequities (Sawhill, 2013; Braveman et al, 2011; Marmot & Wilkinson, 2006; Williams & Collins, 2002).

Hopetown (pseudonym), Mississippi has a population that is 80 percent black and 41 percent of the total population lives below the poverty level (US Census Bureau, 2015). Intergenerational poverty is the norm for many residents of Hopetown whose family legacy is rooted in slavery. Healthy child development requires responsive environments and nurturing relationships that 'build sturdy brain circuits, facilitate emerging capabilities, and strengthen the roots of physical and mental health' (NSCDC, 2012, p.1). The context of daily living for poor children in Hopetown is riddled with multiple challenges that adversely impact their overall development and achievement of their full occupational potential. Many poor children grow up in chaotic, impoverished and unstable family situations in resource-deprived communities thus experiencing chronic stress toxicity. Risk factors that are personal and environmental intersect in complex ways that though not causal, nonetheless increase the magnitude of deprivation and health risk in a manner that is significant and cumulative (Halfon et al, 2014). The biological embedding of adversity and stress coupled with chronic under-stimulation from material and social deprivation undermines the developmental trajectory and leads to problems in learning, behavior and health across the life span (NSCDC, 2012).

High rates of incarceration and deaths due to homicide and disease have widened the gender gap among black Americans (Wolfers et al, 2015). The gender gap and the general disinclination of black men to commit to marriage impact the marriage market and family formation contributing to increasing non-marital births and female-headed families (Charles & Luoh, 2010). Alternate explanations for non-marital childbearing amongst blacks include racial oppression and economic displacement of low class black men (Ricketts, 1989). Compared to other high-income countries, the United States overall has the highest percent of children (27%) being raised by a single parent (Casey & Maldonado, 2012). When it comes to black children, as many as 72% are in single parent homes where mothers live alone or cohabitate; it is not uncommon in Hopetown for a mother to have multiple children with different fathers, who are largely absent. An alternate living arrangement that is also common is grandmother-headed households that appear to have better developmental outcomes for the children (Snyder et al, 2006). A child of a single parent who is low-skilled, unemployed, with little by way of material or social capital experiences chronic and cumulative risk factors that adversely impacts development and occupational potential. The United States ranks the highest for teen births and the state of Mississippi leads the nation in teen pregnancy; a teen in Mississippi is 15 times more likely to give birth compared to a girl in Switzerland (Kearney & Levine, 2012). A child of an adolescent mother is worse off on multiple dimensions of development- physical, economic, cognitive and social dimensions (Amato & Maynard, 2007). Evidence seems to suggest that being on a low economic trajectory, and seeing no prospects for improvement leads teens to have children young (Kearney & Levine, 2012; O'Donohue & Rabin, 1999). This compounds the probability of adolescent mothers dropping out of school, with little or no preparation to participate in the labor market.

Low levels of education, literacy issues, and poor parental attitudes impact the quality and quantity of parents' engagement in child rearing and children's educational activities (McLeod et al, 2014). Economic stressors that put the family at risk for residential instability, food insecurity, and adequate resources to manage daily life stressors negatively impact children's socio-emotional development and well being. Neighborhood violence keeps children indoors thus depriving them of social interactions through play, and these children display a heightened sense of vigilance, mistrust and distrust (Gapen et al, 2011). Children from disadvantaged and segregated neighborhoods also experience social isolation and limited exposure to mainstream social norms, resources, opportunities and role models. This undermines their ability for social integration and participation. Hopetown's public schools, like many in poor neighborhoods, are severely under-resourced, enforce corporal punishment and zero-tolerance policies when dealing with disruptive behaviors in the classroom by dismissing students, relying more on police to arrest children who are placed in juvenile detention facilities (ACLU, 2008). Negative attitudes result in poor black children 'treated as academically deficient and inferior…social deviants and singled out as suspicious or possibly criminal simply because they lived in racialized spaces' (Yull, 2014, p. 9). The 'school to prison pipeline' refers to public policies and practices that push the most vulnerable and at-risk children out of classrooms and into the juvenile and criminal justice systems (ACLU, 2008). Incarceration rates for blacks in general are 6 times higher than whites (Gao, 2014), so much so that incarceration has become 'a new life stage for young, low-skilled black men' (Petit & Western, 2004, p. 151). Increasing rates of incarceration, low education and lack of economic opportunities further increase neighborhood crime and increasing involvement of youth in criminal activities.

In summary, many poor black children in a place like Hopetown grow up experiencing cumulative risk factors with little or no protective factors to alleviate the negative health development trajectory. The problems of residential segregation, under resourced schools, unsafe neighborhoods, high crime rates, lack of economic opportunities and such are structural in nature. While community-driven population based programming will help to a certain degree, addressing the root cause will require macro-level systemic changes to remove structural barriers and boost the protective factors that enhance human development and the occupational potential of the children and the community for full participation.

Toxic stress and early family bonding: Social exclusion from breastfeeding

Breastfeeding provides a practical example for examining how toxic stress may exclude families from occupations that are critical for life course health development. Breastfeeding is an early co-occupation that is protective of health and facilitates infant-mother bonding, yet disparities in breastfeeding behaviors exist and are related to social determinants such as income, level of education, and social support (USDHHS, 2011). Exclusion from breastfeeding, a protective factor, may further compound adversity and contribute to disparities in health outcomes.

Socio-demographics, maternity care practices, postpartum depression, and work or child care environments, among other factors, are known risks for exclusion from breastfeeding (Pitonyak et al 2015; Li et al, 2008). Studies show that younger age, unmarried, primiparous, less education, lower income, participation in the Women, Infants and Children (WIC) supplemental nutrition and education program for low-income mothers, and geographic area are all factors associated with lower rates of initiation and earlier discontinuation of breastfeeding in the U.S. (McDonald et al., 2012; USDHHS, 2011; Guendelman et al., 2009; Li et al., 2005; Li et al., 2008). The identified factors that protect breastfeeding initiation, duration, and exclusivity is associated with higher income, higher education, older age, and being married (USDHHS, 2011; Guendelman et al., 2009). Earlier prenatal care and giving birth in a Baby-Friendly hospital are associated with increased rates of breastfeeding initiation and continuation (Tenfelde et al, 2011; USDHHS, 2011), as are other protective factors such as health insurance, transportation, and employment (Alexander et al, 2002; Kogan et al, 1998). Therefore, participation in this early bonding experience is systematically denied to some families due to toxic stress and other social determinants.

Social determinants and social policy often interact to create early adversity for families leading to a trajectory of decreased occupational potential and family health across the life course (Halfon et al, 2014). Paid parental leave from work enables families to enact early childhood occupations. However federal policy in the United States, the Family and Medical Leave Act (FMLA) (Department of Labor, 2015) creates barriers to early family bonding occupational experiences. For instance, access to paid parental leave and flexible work options are associated with breastfeeding initiation and continuation (Pitonyak et al, 2015; Mirkovic et al, 2014; Jacknowitz, 2008). Lower levels of education and income are associated with risk of not breastfeeding (Johnston & Esposito, 2007). This is not surprising as women with low education and low skills are in employment situations with very limited flexibility, autonomy, and employment benefits. These contextual factors interact to create a nested environment of early adversity for families who also experience early parent-infant separation that has the potential to disrupt early bonding experiences. Many of the working poor qualify for the Federal grants program called Women,

Infants and Children (WIC) as their income level puts them at nutritional risk. A few of the mothers in Hopetown are in the category of the working poor, and a majority receives welfare benefits under the Temporary Assistance for Needy Families (TANF) legislation. These social welfare programs, while well intentioned often have unintended consequences for family life course health development. Simon and Handler (2008) found a negative effect of welfare reform on Medicaid coverage (health insurance for unemployed or low-income individuals) for unmarried mothers, ages 15 to 45 years old, with high school completion or less. They observed that welfare reform increased labor force attachment, but decreased eligibility for Medicaid. The perinatal period is a sensitive time for women's life course health development, so the loss of health insurance places women at increased risk of prenatal and post-birth health conditions. These health conditions may subsequently lead to decreased occupations important for bonding.

Implications for occupational therapy

Current occupational therapy services for children are primarily associated with health insurance or legislation that mandates services for children with disability in educational settings. The Individuals with Disabilities Education Act (IDEA) legislates services for children with disabilities for access to public education (United States Department of Education, 2010). Occupational therapists in these programs primarily address person factors interfering with 'typical' development and occupational performance in the context of education. The cases discussed in this chapter clearly illustrate the large number of children who do not have a disability, but nonetheless are at-risk of not reaching their developmental milestones, their occupational potential, and experiencing social exclusion, on account of structural and contextual factors that reside outside of their control.

The LCHD model is a useful lens for examining the examples of early adversity discussed in this chapter, and their transaction within a nested environment of family, community, and policy contexts. The LCHD model defines the family context as consisting of capacities, process, and caregiving. Adversity from homelessness and lack of family permanency are examples of risk factors within the family context that impact early family routines essential for life course health development and achievement of occupational potential. Chronic poverty and racism can be viewed as risk factors within the LCHD community context, characterized by community assets and accessibility to a care environment; whereas, engagement in early mother-infant bonding occupations, including breast feeding, fits within the LCHD policy context due to the influences of health, social, and work policy.

Table 1 provides some examples of vital roles for preventative occupational therapy in enhancing the occupational potential for children and their families who are experiencing adversity and subsequent social exclusion. The need for occupational therapy to go beyond direct, impairment-based intervention has been shown by the cases. The profession can work with families, communities, and advocate for changes in social and health policy. A unique contribution that occupational therapy can make for addressing these unmet needs and public policy is building the research evidence on the long-term effects of toxic stress and occupational injustices on the health development trajectory, and subsequent risk for social exclusion and diminished participation.

Table 1
Potential roles for occupational therapists to promote healthy child development

Enhancing occupational potential of children: • Interventions targeting emotional self-regulation, appropriate behavioral responses, interpersonal communication skills and incorporated into play may help improve the developmental trajectory and may also reinforce positive socialization and appropriate classroom behaviors.   • Establish context stability and structure to cultivate (1) healthy occupational habits and routines (Groza & Ileana, 1996; Lin et al, 2005; Hopper et al, 2010); (2) occupational skills and behaviors. For example, communication (Hwa-Froelich & Matsuo, 2010; Ellesoff, 2013); social interactions (Tarullo et al, 2007); occupational performance in academic and school context (Vorria, et al, 2006)
Enhancing the occupational potential of caregivers: • Parent education to enhance caregiving capacities to understand and manage difficult behaviors; (Townsend & McWhirter, 2005); strategies to set up daily routines, stress management, etc. (Paul Ward, 2009; Tirella et al, 2012)   • Reinforce caregiver-child co-occupations to enhance bonding within family daily routines such as early reciprocal communication for increased language (NSCDC, 2015); and early reading which can foster self-regulation and may be protective for later school achievement (Masten et al, 2014)
Community-level services: • After-school programs that use play to enhance social skills, self-esteem, gross and fine motor skills can be provided in collaboration with school systems, parks and recreation services, and welfare support services.   • Providing screenings and services in shelters, supported housing, and primary care (Allen et al, 2010).   • Consulting with organizations and communities to create environments (physical and social) and routines supportive of family occupation. For example, clean spaces for breastfeeding in workplaces and day care centers.
Advocacy & Public policy: • Advocacy for change in social policy that constrain desired family routines. For example, paid parental leave to promote family occupations that foster emotional development of child.   • Context stability and permanency in family life including housing, transportation and custodial care.   • Early access to services to address self-regulation, skill development, parent education, etc. Advocating for affordable and accessible enhanced EI Programs in shelters, supported housing, and primary care (Allen et al, 2010).   • Influence public policy that addresses contextual and structural risk factors and promote policy that fosters protective factors to create conditions that favor a positive life-course health development trajectory.

A critique of occupational therapy practice in the United States is that a majority of occupational therapists are in biomedical settings and practice is tied to reimbursement through the healthcare industry (Gupta & Taff, 2015). About 2% of occupational therapists identify as community-based practitioners although it is unclear if they are associated with the delivery of social services (AOTA, 2015). There are a number of social service sectors where occupational therapy can meet the occupational needs of some of society's most vulnerable, such as the systems that deal with welfare, incarceration, unemployment. The profession has a social responsibility to influence policies that create structural barriers to engagement in health promoting occupations for all, and minimize the early adversity experiences that in the long run impact societal health.

Conclusion

Occupational potential is dynamic and, starting in childhood, develops over one's entire lifetime (Wicks, 2005). Fulfilling one's occupational potential is necessary for health and living a meaningful life. Those who are experience occupational injustices are unable to reach their occupational potential and therefore cannot experience self-efficacy and the transforming power of occupational engagement (Christiansen, 2000; Townsend, 1997). Social and institutional conditions instigate the path to occupational injustices and social exclusion and the accompanying loss of meaning, motivation, and self-efficacy. However, being part of a community of occupationally engaged persons can minimize social exclusion and allow persons and communities to more freely pursue their occupational potential. As demonstrated in this chapter, the LCHD model offers an approach where early adversity and social exclusion can be addressed in transdisciplinary and population-based ways centered on enabling health-promoting occupations. Whether the source of adversity is lack of opportunities to experience family bonding, a nurturing and stable family/home (ie: foster care/ institutionalization or homelessness), residential and racial segregation, health and occupational inequities can be minimized through a combination of occupation-based programs, just and ethical policies that link lives in pursuit of achieving optimal occupational potential.

References

Alexander, G. R, Kogan, M. D, and Nabukera, S. (2002) Racial differences in prenatal care use in the United States: Are disparities decreasing? *Research and Practice*, 92, 12, 1970 -1975. doi:10.2105/AJPH.92.12.1970

Alexander, J.M. (2008) *Capabilities and Social Justice: The political philosophy of Amartya Sen and Martha Nussbaum*. Aldershot: Ashgate

Allen, S.G, Berry, A.D., Juanona, A.B, Chalasani, R.K. and Mack, P.K. (2010) Enhancing developmentally oriented primary care: An Illinois initiative to increase developmental screening in medical homes. *Pediatrics*, 126, S160-164

American Occupational Therapy Association, (2015) Salary and workforce survey. [Accessed

5 October 2015 at http://www.aota.org/-/media/Corporate/Files/Secure/Educations-Careers/Salary-Survey/2015-AOTA-Workforce-Salary-Survey-LOW-RES.pdf]

Anda, R.F., Felitti, V.J, Bremner, J.D, Walker, Ch., J.D Whitfield, C., Perry, B.D., Dube, S. R., and Giles, W.H. (2006) The enduring effects of abuse and related adverse experiences in childhood. *European Archives of Psychiatry and Clinical Neuroscience*, 256, 3, 174-186

Amato, P. R., and Maynard, R. A. (2007) Decreasing nonmarital births and strengthening marriage to reduce poverty. *The Future of Children*, 17,2,117-141.

American Civil Liberties Union (2008) *Locating the School-to-Prison Pipeline*. [Accessed 19 November 2014 at https://www.aclu.org/sites/default/files/images/asset_upload_file966_35553.pdf]

Beckes, L., Ijerzman, H., and Tops, M. (2015) Toward a radically embodied neuroscience of attachment and relationships. *Frontiers of Human Neuroscience*, 9, 266

Braveman, P. A., Kumanyika, S., Fielding, J., LaVeist, T., Borrell, L. N., Manderscheid, R., and Troutman, A. (2011) Health disparities and health equity: The issue is justice. *American Journal of Public Health*, 10, S1, S149-S155

Bassuk, E., De Candia, C., Beach C. and Berman, F. (2014) *America's Youngest Outcasts. A report card on child homelessness*. Waltham. MA. National Center on Family Homelessness at American Institutes for Research. [Accessed 12 March 2015 at http://www.homelesschildrenamerica.org/mediadocs/280.pdf]

Bassuk, E., Richard, M. K. and Tsertsvadze, A. (2015) The prevalence of mental illness in homeless children: A systematic review and meta-analysis. *Clinical Keys*, 54, 2, 86-96.e2

Casey, T., and Maldonado, L. (2012) *Worst Off: Single-parent families in the United States. A cross-national comparison of single parenthood in the US and sixteen other high-income countries*. New York, NY: Legal Momentum, the Women's Legal Defense and Education Fund

Charles, K.K. and Luoh, M.C. (2010) Male incarceration, the marriage market, and female outcomes. *Review of Economics and Statistics*, 92, 3, 614-627

Christiansen, C. (2000) Identity, personal projects and happiness: Self construction in everyday action. *Journal of Occupational Science*, 7, 3, 98-107

Centers for Disease Control and Prevention (2013) *CDC Health disparities and inequalities report - United States, 2013*. [Accessed 2 March 2015 at http://www.cdc.gov/mmwr/pdf/other/su6203.pdf]

Cutuli, J. J. and Herbers, J. E.(2014) Promoting resilience for children who experience family homelessness: Opportunities to encourage developmental competence. *Cityscape*, 16, 113-139

Diamond, A. and Lee, L. (2011) Interventions shown to aid executive function development in children 4-12 years old. *Science* 333, 959-964

Drury, S.S., Theall, K., Gleason, M.M., Smyke, A.T., DeVivo, I., Wong, Y.Y., Fox, N.A., Zeanah, C.H. and Nelson, C.A. (2012) Telomere length and early severe social deprivation: Linking early adversity to cellular aging. *Molecular Psychiatry*, 17,719-727

Duncan, G., Ziol-Guest, K.M. and Kalil, A. (2010) Early childhood poverty and adult attainment, behavior and health. *Child Development*, 65, 2, 296-318

Forkey, H. and Szilagyi, M. (2014) Foster care and healing from complex childhood trauma. *Pediatric Clinics of North America*, 61, 1059-1072

Gao, G. (2014) *Chart Of The Week: The black-white gap in incarceration rates*. [Accessed 10 January, 2015 at http://www.pewresearch.org/fact-tank/2014/07/18/chart-of-the-week-the-black-white-gap-in-incarceration-rates/]

Gapen, M., Cross, D., Ortigo, K., Graham, A., Johnson, E., Evces, M., Ressler, K. J. and Bradley,

B. (2011), Perceived neighborhood disorder, community cohesion, and PTSD symptoms among low-income African Americans in an urban health setting. *American Journal of Orthopsychiatry*, 81, 31–37. doi: 10.1111/j.1939-0025.2010.01069.x

Gronski, M. P., Bogan, K. E., Kloeckner, J., Russell-Thomas, D., Taff, S. D., Walker, K. A., and Berg, C. (2013) Childhood toxic stress: A community role in health promotion for occupational therapists. *American Journal of Occupational Therapy*, 67, 6, e148-e153

Groza, V. and Ileana, D. (2006) A follow up study of adopted children from Romania. *Child and Adolescent Social Work Journal*, 13, 6, 542-565

Guendelman, S., Kosa, J. L., Pearl, M., Graham, S., Goodman, J., and Kharrazi, M. (2009) Juggling work and breastfeeding: Effects of maternity leave and occupational characteristics. *Pediatrics*, 123,e38

Gupta, J., and Taff, S. D. (2015). The illusion of client-centred practice. *Scandinavian Journal of occupational therapy*, 22,4, 244-251

Halfon, N., Berkowitz, G. and Klee, L. (1992) Children in foster care in California: An examination of Medicaid reimbursed health services utilization. *Pediatrics*, 89, 1230-1237

Halfon, N. & Forrest, C. B. (2018). The emerging theoretical framework of life course health development. In N. Halfon, C. B. Forrest, R. M. Lerner & E. M Faustman (Eds.) *Handbook of life course health development* .(19-46). Cham, Switzerland: Springer

Halfon, N. and Hochstein, M. (2002). Life course health development: An integrated framework for developing health, policy, and research. *The Milbank Quarterly*, 80, 3, 433-479

Halfon, N., Larson, K., Lu, M., Tullis, E., and Russ, S. (2014) Lifecourse health development: Past, present and future. *Maternal Child Health Journal*, 18, 344-365

Herbers, J. E., Cutuli, M. J., Supkoff, L., Narayan, A. J, and Masten, A. S. (2014) Parenting and Co-regulation: Adaptive systems for competence in children experiencing homelessness. *American Journal of Orthopsychiatry*, 84, 420-430

Hopper. E.K., Bassuk, E. and Oliver, J. (2010) Trauma-informed care in homelessness services settings. *The Open Health Services and Policies Journal*, 3, 80-100

Hwa-Froelich, D. A. and Matsuo, H. (2010). Communication development and differences in children adopted from China and Eastern Europe. *Language, Speech, and Hearing Services in Schools*, 4, 3, 349-366

Jacknowitz, A. (2008) The role of workplace characteristics in breastfeeding practices. *Women and Health*, 47, 2, 87-111

Jee, S.H., Conn, J.M. and Nilsen, W.J. et al. (2008) Learning difficulties among children separated from a parent. *Ambulatory Pediatrics*, 8, 3, 63-8

Johnston, M. L. and Esposito, N. (2007) Barriers and facilitators for breastfeeding among working women in the United States. *Journal of Obstetric, Gynecologic, and Neonatal Nursing*, 36, 1, 9-20

Kearney, M. S. and Levine, P. B. (2012) *Why is the teen birth rate in the United States so high and why does it matter?* (No. w17965). National Bureau of Economic Research

Kogan, M., Martin, J., Alexander, G., Kotelchuck, M., Ventura, S. and Frigoletto, F. (1998) The changing pattern of prenatal care utilization in the United States, 1981-1995, using different prenatal care indices. *JAMA*, *279*, 20, 1623-1628

Lin, S. H., Cermak, S., Coster, W. J. and Laurie Miller, L. (2005) The relation between length of institutionalization and sensory integration in children adopted from Eastern Europe. *American Journal of Occupational Therapy*, 59, 2, 139-147

Lombardi, J., Mosle, A., Pate, N., Schumacher, R. and Stedron, J. (2014) *Gateways to two generations: The potential for early childhood programs and partnerships to support children and parents together*. [Accessed 12 March 2015 at http://ascend.aspeninstitute.org/pages/gateways-to-two-generations]

Marmot, M. and Wilkinson, R. (2006). *Social determinants of health*. New York, NY: Oxford University Press

Masten, A. S., Cutuli, J. J., Herbers, J. E., Hinz, E., Obradovic, J. and Wenzel, A. J. (2014) Academic risk and resilience in the context of homelessness. *Child Development Perspectives*, 8, 4, 201-206

McDonald, S. D., Pullenayegum, E., Chapman, B., Vera, C., Giglia, L., Fusch, C. and Foster, G. (2012) Prevalence and predictors of exclusive breastfeeding at hospital discharge. *Obstetrics and Gynecology*, 119, 6, 1171-1179

McKinney-Vento Homeless Assistance Act, 42 U.S.C. § 1032 (2002, 2010)

McLeod, V., Mistry, R.S. and Hardaway, C.R. (2014) Poverty and children's development: Familial processes as mediating influences. in E.T. Gershoff, R.S .Mistry and D.A. Crosby (eds), *Societal context of child development*. New York, NY: Oxford University Press

Mekonnen, R., Noonan, K. and Rubin, D. (2009) Achieving better health care outcomes for children in foster care. *Pediatric Clinics of North America*, 56, 405-415

Mirkovic, K. R., Perrine, C. G., Scanlon, K. S. and Grummer-Strawn, L. M. (2014) Maternity leave duration and full-time/part-time work status are associated with US mothers' ability to meet breastfeeding intentions. *Journal of Human Lactation*, 30, 4, 416-419. doi:10.1177/0890334414543522

Moodie, S. and Ramos, M. (2014) Culture counts: Engaging Black and Latino parents of young children in family support programs. *Child Trends*. [Accessed 22 March 2015 at http://www.childtrends.org/wp-content/uploads/2014/10/2014-44BCultureCountsFullReport.pdf]

National Scientific Council on the Developing Child (2015) *Supportive relationships and active skill building strengthen the foundations of resilience*. Working paper #13. [Accessed 22 March 2015 at http://www.developingchild.harvard.edu]

National Scientific Council on the Developing Child. (2012) *The Science of Neglect: The persistent absence of responsive care disrupts the developing brain*. Working Paper 12. [Accessed 6 February 2015 at http://www.developingchild.harvard.edu]

National Scientific Council on the Developing Child (2010) *Early experiences can alter gene expression and affect long-term development*. Working Paper 10 [Accessed 16 December 2015 at http://www.developingchild.harvard.edu]

National Scientific Council on the Developing Child (2005) *Excessive stress disrupts the architecture of the developing brain*. Working paper 3. [Accessed 30 March 2015 at http://www.developingchild.harvard.edu]

O'Donoghue, T. and Rabin, M. (1999) Doing it now or later. *American Economic Review* 89, 1, 103–124

Paul-Ward, A. (2009) Social and occupational justice barriers in the transition to adulthood from foster care, *American Journal of Occupational Therapy*, 63, 81-88

Pecora, P. J., Kessler, R. C., O'Brien, K., White, C. R., Williams, J., Hiripi, E. and Herrick, M. A. (2006) Educational and employment outcomes of adults formerly placed in foster care: Results from the Northwest Foster Care Alumni Study. *Children and Youth Services Review*, 28, 12, 1459-1481. doi:10.1016/j.childyouth.2006.04.003

Pitonyak, J. S., Gupta, J., Pergolotti, M. (2020). Health Policy Perspectives: Understanding policy influences on health and occupation through the use of the life course health development (LCHD) framework. *American Journal of Occupational Therapy*, 74, 1–6. https://doi.

org/10.5014/ajot.2020.742002

Pitonyak, J. S., Mroz, T. M. and Fogelberg, D. (2015) Expanding client-centred thinking to include social determinants: A practical scenario based on the occupation of breastfeeding. *Scandinavian Journal of Occupational Therapy*, 22, 4, 277-82

Pitonyak, J. S., Souza, K., Umeda, C., & Jirikowic, T. (2021). Using a health promotion approach to frame parent experiences of family routines and the significance for health and well-being. *Journal of Occupational Therapy, Schools, & Early Intervention*. DOI: 10.1080/19411243.2021.1983499

Ricketts, E. (1989) The origin of black female-headed families. *Focus*, 12, 1, 32-36.

Rosenberg, S. A., Zhang, D. and Robinson, C. (2008) Prevalence of developmental delays and participation in early intervention services for young children. *Pediatrics*, 12, e1503-1509

Rybski, D. and Wilder, E. (2008). A pilot study to identify developmental delay in children in underserved community child care. *Journal of Allied Health, 37(1)*, e34-49

Sawhill, I.V. (2013) Family structure: Growing importance of class. [Accessed 24 January 2015 at http://www.brookings.edu/research/articles/2013/01/family-structure-class-sawhill]

Shonkoff, J. P. (2012). Leveraging the biology of adversity to address the roots of disparities in health and development. *Proceedings of the National Academy of Sciences*, 109 (Suppl. 2), 17302–17307. [Accessed 17 September 2014 at http://dx.doi.org/10.1073/pnas.1121259109]

Simon, K. I. and Handler, A. (2008). Welfare reform and insurance coverage during the pregnancy period: Implications for preconception and interconception care. *Women's Health Issues*, 18S, S97-S106

Smith, P. H., Coley, S. L., Labbok, M. H., Cupito, S. and Nwokah, E. (2012). Early breastfeeding experiences of adolescent mothers: a qualitative prospective study. *International breastfeeding journal*, 7, 1, 13

Snyder, A. R., McLaughlin, D. K. and Findeis, J. (2006) Household composition and poverty among female-headed households with children: Differences by race and residence. *Rural Sociology*, 71,4, 597-624

Tarullo, A. R., Bruce, J. and Gunnar, M. R. (2007) False belief and emotion understanding in post-institutionalized children. *Social Development*, 16,1, 57-78

Taussig, H., Culhane, S., Garrido, E. and Knudtson, M. (2012) RCT of a mentoring and skills group program: Placement and permanency outcomes for foster youth. *Pediatrics*, 130, 1, e33-e39

Tirella, L, Tickle-Degnen, L., Miller, L. and Bedell, G. (2012) Parent strategies for addressing the needs of their newly adopted child. *Physical and Occupational Therapy in Pediatrics*, 32, 1:97–110

Tenfelde, S., Finnegan, L. and Hill, P. D. (2011) Predictors of breastfeeding exclusivity in a WIC sample. *JOGNN*, 40, 2, 179-189

Townsend, E. (1997). Occupation: Potential for personal and social transformation. *Journal of Occupational Science*, 4, 1, 18-26

Townsend, K. C. and McWhirter, B. T. (2005). Connectedness: A review of the literature with implications for counseling, assessment, and research. *Journal of Counseling and Development: JCD*, 83, 2, 191

U.S. Census Bureau (2015). *State and County Quick Facts*. [Accessed 5 April 2015 at http://quickfacts.census.gov/qfd/states/28/28027.html]

U.S. Department of Education. (2010). *Thirty-five years of progress in educating children with disabilities through IDEA*. [Accessed 17 January 2016 at http://www2.ed.gov/about/offices/

list/osers/idea35/history/idea-35-history.pdf]

U. S. Department of Health and Human Services (USDHHS). (2011). *The Surgeon General's Call to Action to Support Breastfeeding.* Washington, DC: USDHHS, Office of the Surgeon General. [Accessed 10 January 2015 at http://www.surgeongeneral.gov/library/calls/breastfeeding/calltoactiontosupportbreastfeeding.pdf]

U. S. Department of Labor. (2015). *Family and Medical Leave Act.* [Accessed 24 April 2015 at http://www.dol.gov/whd/fmla/]

Vorria, P., Papaligoura, Z., Sarafidou, J., Kopakaki, M., Dunn, J., Van Ijzendoorn, M. and Kontopoulou, A. (2006) The development of adopted children after institutional care: A follow-up study. *Journal of Child Psychology and Psychiatry,* 47,12, 1246-53

Wicks, A. (2005) Understanding occupational potential. *Journal of Occupational Science,* 12, 3, 130-139

Williams D.R. and Collins C. (2002) US socioeconomic and racial differences in health: patterns and explanations. in T.A. LaVeist (Ed.). *A Public Health Reader: Race, Ethnicity and Health.* John Wiley and Sons (pp.391-431)

Whiteford, G.E. and Pereira, R. B. (2012) Occupation, inclusion and participation. in G.E. Whiteford and C. Hocking (Eds). *Occupational science: Society, inclusion, participation.* Hoboken, New Jersey: Wiley-Blackwell (pp.187-207)

Wolfers, J., Leonhardt, D. and Quealy, K. (2015) *1.5 Million Missing Black Men.* [Accessed 20 April 2015 at http://www.nytimes.com/interactive/2015/04/20/upshot/missing-black-men.html?rref=upshotandabt=0002andabg=0]

Yull, D. G. (2014) Race has always mattered: an intergeneration look at race, space, place, and educational experiences of blacks. *Education Research International,* Article ID 683035, 13 pages, [Accessed 7 March 2015 at http://dx.doi.org/10.1155/2014/683035]

Chapter 3
Understanding the relationship between occupation and social inclusion of blind and visually impaired (BVI) people in conservative Malaysian Chinese families with the Kawa Model

Jou Yin Teoh, Alvin Ng Lai Oon, and Michael Iwama

People who are blind are typically seen as being disabled and dependent on others in daily activities. Being seen this way often results in being marginalized and excluded from most social activities. With regard to traditional Chinese thinking, people who are less able tend to be pitied and are kept marginalised fwrom the mainstream society. Given that one of the purposes of occupational therapy is to facilitate social inclusion of disabled people, it is important to have cultural competency in addressing these social issues in order to bridge the gaps preventing the blind from assimilating into society. As such, this chapter explores the concept of social inclusion within conservative West Malaysian Chinese families for people who are blind and visually impaired (BVI) through a case study which was part of registered research under Universiti Kebangsaan Malaysia (Teoh, 2011). Further, the chapter explicates how their inclusion or exclusion within the family can be linked to their participation and engagement in daily activities (otherwise known as occupations).

To contextualise this chapter's discussion, a short introduction on Malaysia and its cultural make-up is described with regards to how this chapter's exploration of Chinese cultural dynamics is justified as part of advancement of practices in Malaysian occupational therapy. This then flows into a description of how an Asian occupational therapy practice framework -the Kawa (River) Model (Iwama, 2006) can be used to better understand how social inclusion for the BVI people can be facilitated through occupational therapy.

The Chinese in Malaysia: A brief history and current situation

Malaysia is a South East Asian country, comprising two segments: West Malaysia, and East Malaysia which forms part of the island of Borneo. Prior to the formation of Malaysia as a country, West Malaysia was known as the Federation of Malaya while the states of East Malaysia were known as the Crown Colony of North Borneo and the Crown Colony of Sarawak respectively. Malaysia has a population of about 28 million, out of which 22.5 million live in West Malaysia and 5.72 million live in East Malaysia (Department of Statistics Malaysia, 2010). The people of Malaysia come from various cultural and ethnic backgrounds, with Malays forming the dominant ethnic community accounting for 50.1% of the population, followed by the Malaysian Chinese (22.6%), Malaysian Indians (6.7%) and indigenous people such as the Kadazan-Dusun, Murut, Bidayuh, Iban, Penan, or Senoi; and other groups such as Malaysian Siamese and Kristang (Malacca Portuguese, descendants of intermarriages between Portuguese colonisers and local Asian people) that make up the remainder of the population (Central Intelligence Agency, 2015).

The development of the ethnic Chinese community in Malaysia differs according to geographic location and when the emigration occurred. The West Malaysian Chinese community developed in a distinctly different manner from the ethnic Chinese people in East Malaysia due to the differences in cultural and ethnic composition of both areas. This chapter focuses specifically on the lived experiences of the ethnic Chinese community whose ancestors immigrated into Malaya before its independence from British rule in 1957.

The Kawa Model is comprised of the following four interrelated constructs:

- *River Flow* (main life priorities). In this instance, the River Flow is used to represent the main life priorities of conservative Malaysian Chinese families and how they influence the life experiences of their BVI family members.
- *River Banks* (environments – physical, social, virtual, cultural), representing the cultural environments which Malaysian Chinese people inhabit (both BVI and non-BVI).
- *Driftwood* (influencing factors – factors that can influence the river flow to be either positive or negative, depending on circumstances), representing cultural perspectives that can either encourage social inclusion or lead to social exclusion.
- *Rocks* (obstacles and challenges), specifically towards social inclusion of BVI people within the conservative Malaysian Chinese family.

Studying the dynamic relationship between these four constructs potentially allows us to gain an understanding of how social inclusion can be facilitated, resulting in a fifth construct known as *spaces*. The spaces are points within the framework of the river that can be manipulated to facilitate changes to the other structures (such as widening the river banks or breaking a rock) which would expand spaces in the river to allow greater 'flow' of social inclusion, as well as increased participation and engagement in occupations.

River Flow: 'Face' and how it influences social inclusion for BVI people within the conservative Malaysian Chinese family

To understand the phenomenon of social inclusion for BVI people within conservative Malaysian Chinese families, besides the personal narratives of BVI people themselves, we also draw upon understanding of parenting, socio-emotional child development, language and education, spirituality and traditional beliefs, coping and illness behaviours, constructions of disability, and a variety of other factors that constitute the Malaysian Chinese lived experience. However, as anthropological, sociological and psychosocial research specific to the Malaysian Chinese population is significantly limited, we also draw upon perspectives from Hong Kong, China and Taiwan, places with a predominantly ethnic Chinese population which share significant cultural commonalities with the more conservative, Chinese-educated Malaysian Chinese (as detailed in the *river banks* section of this chapter). There is even less literature on the experience of BVI within the context of Malaysian Chinese experiences, so further research needs to be conducted in order to gain a better understanding of this area.

Teoh (2011) indicated that feelings of social exclusion within the family were expressed in narratives among Malaysian Chinese BVI people. We will base this chapter on the narratives of S, a blind Malaysian Chinese man in his 40s who belonged to a conservative family but has now moved out to live on his own. It is important to note that this interview was conducted in English and the respondent's narratives are reported verbatim in colloquial Malaysian English.

> *'When I small that time ah, I because my parents are, when this year my parents they all ask them to hide in the, I mean ask them to hide in the room. We also human, they also human, right or not? Only the thing is we cannot see only, right or not. So it's what do you call, no good isn't it?'*

S describes being socially isolated by his family out of shame and embarrassment. This is very much linked to the social construct known in Chinese as 'face'.

According to Ho (1976, p.883):

> 'Face is the respectability and/or deference which a person can claim for himself from others, by virtue of the relative position he occupies in his social network and the degree to which he is judged to have functioned adequately in that position as well as acceptably in his general conduct; the face extended to a person by others is a function of the degree of congruence between judgments of his total condition in life, including his actions as well as those of people closely associated with him, and the social expectations that others have placed upon him. In terms of two interacting parties, face is the reciprocated compliance, respect, and/or deference that each party expects from, and extends to, the other party.'

Therefore face can be described as the governing force for guiding social interactions and also a way to determine one's position and status in society. Face originates from the Confucian emphasis on harmony within the social order of the clan. Maintaining face is essential for the maintenance of harmony, and parents of disabled children might regard having a BVI child as a 'loss of face', disruptive to the family's position in society. There are essentially two factors that influence whether face is enhanced or threatened: morality and achievements or capability. The perceived status of one's achievements also influences the extent of the loss or gain of face. Chu (1991) found that moral episodes are more likely to cause a sense of loss of face than episodes concerning one's capability or status. Therefore the primary reason why S's family hides him away from visitors could be to preserve the face of the rest of his family members from judgements of morality, and not necessarily with the intention to socially exclude him because of his blindness.

The association between congenital BVI and a family's loss of moral face developed from a combination of Confucian culture and Buddhism. According to the Buddhist Law of Cause and Effect, congenital disabilities and birth defects can represent the consequences of misdeeds in past lives, therefore they can be perceived as an indication of a lack of morality which is associated with face (Hwang & Han, 2010). This perceived lack of morality would not be limited to the child alone, but also extended to the child's family in line with collectivist Confucian culture.

The idea that the behaviour of S's family is due to the need to protect his other family members from losing moral face is in line with the Confucian ideals of 'sacrificing the 'smaller self' for the good of the 'larger self''. Hwang & Han (2010) suggest that in Confucianism, individual lives (the smaller self) are a continuation of their parents' and ancestors' lives. Thus it is likely to include family members in the territory of one's self (the larger self) therefore allowing them to be especially liable to the feelings of having glory or shame together under the construction of the greater self. Based on this understanding, we now know that S's feelings of face and personal self-worth were regarded as less important than the face of the larger self of family members.

Interestingly, S's perceived exclusion within his family in the presence of visitors did not necessarily affect his participation in occupations. Even though S expresses anger at his family for hiding him away from the presence of visitors as a child, he expresses gratitude that his family actually allowed him to attend residential school and even brought him along for outings during school holidays:

> 'Ok, definitely want to thank my parents, to can allow me to go to school and umm, thanks all the relatives all lah, my grandmother they all ok – they're not around ah. My mother also, my father… My father still around lah. My mother is no more already so I thank them to bringing me up and to allow me to go to school.
>
> My father just go to school just visit me in school. My grandfather that time when I primary school he always visit me in school also. My father just visit me when I secondary school that time lah. Every Sunday go visit me in school and then sometimes when school holiday also they bring me out here and there.'

This could be linked to the secondary factor that influences face, which is achievement, which we will expand upon later in the driftwood segment.

S describes family life after he left home to go to boarding school as shown below, indicating that he prefers to spend his time away from home and family because 'there is nothing to do':

> 'I seldom go home actually. Oh because when after school like after work like now during holiday time when I go back I also feel like nothing to do ah, quite bored ah. Cuz seriously speaking all this honestly speaking ah, I go home nothing to do because I go home just go back and then I listen to radio and besides listen to radio I go and hide in their room lah. And sleep in their room and all those lah.'

River Banks: The conservative Malaysian Chinese family: how they fit into the Malaysian Chinese community and how family background can relate to the experience of being blind

Taking some time to understand the school systems of Malaysian Chinese people can give us better insight into influences on their thinking and behaviour. There is a Chinese saying that 'regardless of how poor one gets, one cannot be poor in education'. This reflects how highly Chinese society regards education.

There are two rather distinct groups of Chinese immigrants to Malaya. The first group established their presence in Malaya from as early as the 15th century (West, 2009) and thus have had more opportunities over time to be assimilated into the local culture. Assimilation also meant they were more likely to adopt English education and a more Westernised / cosmopolitan outlook. The trend of Chinese families of sending children to English-medium schools persisted up until the 1960s because acquiring an English education was perceived to be of material advantage (Lee, 2000). English medium schools are open to everyone regardless of ethnicity (Wong et. al, 2012) and provide students with intercultural circumstances in which participants are able to learn how to retain the sense of their original ethnic identity in a multicultural setting using a language that is not native to their original culture (Lee, 2003). Malaysian researchers have found that ability to use English well is not necessarily linked to any erosion of ethnic identity (Wong et. al., 2012; Lee, 2003) and that Malaysians in general are able to maintain distinct elements of their original ethnic identity while using the exposure to other languages as a resource. DeBernardi (2004) states that even during the colonial period, traditional practices were still very popular even among English educated Chinese and that new forms and meanings for Chinese traditional culture had started to develop within the contexts of colonialism, globalisation, modernisation and nationalism.

The second group emigrated into Malaya in the late 18th to early 20th century and worked as coolies (hard labourers), but they had a tradition of entrepreneurship and saved up enough money over time to start and run their own businesses, establish Chinese schools and prosper in their new homeland (Carstens, 2005). Due to their Chinese-educated family background, they tend to be more traditional in their outlook than their English educated brethren. Chinese-medium schools originally started out with a very homogenous population, and according to Goh (2012) learning materials were typically based on classics from China, with the added study of abacus and calligraphy. Each Chinese school had their own unique choices of teaching materials, with some schools even going to the extent of making their own to suit their context (Goh, 2012). What one Chinese school does, others do not necessarily follow and there was no standardised system. There was a shift over time however, from a very China-oriented system - history studies with China as a focal point and holidays to celebrate the birthdays of Sun Yat-Sen and to honour Confucius - to one that was more oriented to living in Malaya (Tan, 1997).

Over time these two distinct groups have evolved into both ends of a spectrum with varying levels of adherence to the original culture, beliefs and values of Chinese tradition in between.

All formal education for BVI people however, has been carried out first in the

English-medium, then later in Malay-medium national schools (Reddy & Tan, 2001). Formal education for BVI people started in 1926 with the St. Nicholas' Home for the Blind, established by Anglican missionaries (Denison & Ooi, 1994) and any further development was completely led by Christian community groups and religious institutions up until 1948 when the Princess Elizabeth School for the Blind was established, signifying the start of the government's formal involvement in special education (Nordin, 2001). Integrated programmes which placed classes for special needs children within mainstream schools were initiated in 1981 as an alternative to residential schools which catered exclusively for special needs children which was the norm previously (Nordin, 2001). There are six residential special education government schools in Malaysia that cater exclusively for the blind – three primary schools in West Malaysia (in Penang, Johor, Kuala Lumpur); one primary school in Kuching, Sarawak; and one primary school in Tuaran, Sabah; and one secondary school in Kuala Lumpur for the whole country (Reddy & Tan, 2001). As far as we know, there has been no research conducted to date that explores how this form of school system has influenced the cultural and ethnic identities of BVI people in the Malaysian Chinese community.

As studies on Westernised Chinese people in urban areas show departure from traditional beliefs and more adoption and assimilation of Western attitudes (Lee & Tan, 2000; Tan, et al., 2005), further research needs to be conducted to determine whether these differences of attitudes within members of a family would contribute to a divide between BVI people educated in more Westernised / cosmopolitan systems and their more conservative families, leading to feelings of social exclusion at the family level. Based on existing studies about the Malaysian Chinese community but not specific to BVI people, this divide exists. The exclusion of those from English / national school educated backgrounds by their Chinese-educated and more conservative counterparts is more apparent when the former is seen to be less proficient in their mother tongue (Lee 2003, 2005; Wong et. al., 2012), therefore it can be inferred that there is a possibility the same could apply for BVI Malaysian Chinese as well. Further exploration of this area is needed.

Driftwood: How do occupations enhance face and subsequently social inclusion within the family?

In Chinese culture, face can be enhanced or threatened by the success or failure of the pursuit of certain life goals. Hwang (2012, p.247) calls these goals 'achievement goals' and classifies them according to the following terms: 'goals of vertical distinctiveness (VD goals)', 'personal goals', and 'goals of horizontal distinctiveness (HD goals)'. He defines them as follows:

- VD goals are life goals highly valued by society. Attaining these goals generally implies a victory through severe competition and a high degree of social appraisal.
- Personal goals are goals pursued by a determined individual because of one's personal interest. The reason for pursuing this type of goal is due to one's intrinsic motivation which is irrelevant to any extrinsic reward.
- HD goals are goals which might be valued by one's peer group but not necessarily

by the rest of society. HD goals can be regarded as an extension of personal goals.

Out of these three types of goals, VD goals are the ones most likely to cause one's elders - parents and teachers - to gain or lose face (Liang et. al., 2007). Wang & Chang (2010) also found that parents were more likely to support their children in the achievement of VD goals rather than HD goals. Han (2013) conducted further research in this area with Taiwanese parents and her findings about parental expectations for their children were congruent with Huang's theory, with the additional attribute of 'good behaviour' besides achievement of goals. This fits in with our earlier discussions in the *river* segment about face and morality, indicating that even if one fails to achieve VD or HD goals, social acceptable conduct in terms of how one carries oneself while performing the activities that lead to these goals is still highly valued.

Achievement is defined by the Merriam-Webster online dictionary as 'something that has been done or achieved through effort: a result of hard work.' As a doing word, achievement goals can therefore be associated with the term known to some in the Western world as occupations. Based on this understanding, we can assume that engaging and performing well in VD occupations would enhance the face of S's family and contribute to better harmony both for the family and within the family, whereas the inability to engage in them (or to a lesser extent, failure to perform) can result in further loss of face and subsequently even disharmony.

Let us take a look at some of the occupations that S describes as being particularly significant to him and also examine whether they are in line with VD and face:

Education

'(GRANDMOTHER) Last time when she want to bring me to school, she go to welfare, go to doctor, ask the doctor to write letter, so need to go welfare. Bring me to welfare, bring me to doctor. And then when I got to school also she still bring me to hostel, bring to school, send me to school, together with my family. She very good lah, because last time she take care of me very well actually eh.

That I am proud of I mean I can study until ok lah, I mean not until University lah, but at least I got a job. At least I can study until – what do you call? Until Form 5, until whatever lah. I mean uhh is a good enough also. In the same time I think that got people also is more ... I mean ar, some of them don't have study and all those er, so that is what I am proud of lah.'

Education and academic achievement is prized among the Chinese community worldwide. There is a Chinese saying 'regardless of how poor one gets, one cannot be poor in education' which reflects the value and regard Chinese society has for education. Education has traditionally been regarded as the one and only means of social mobility since the times of Imperial China (Cheng & Wong, 1996) hence it continues to maintain high VD in Chinese society until today. As we can see from S's narratives, his family – most notably his grandmother who was his primary caretaker – was very supportive towards his education.

Independent living

'My mother also as well also lah. Coz when I go to school, after school and I ... She got,

she taught me this and that. Yeah, do a lot house work you know. That one must mention, my mother.

Ok lah like bathing all this like personal care like bathing all these things I ... of course I can bathe myself la. Feeding ok no problem what. And then uhh its like normal people and then uhhh like washing ... Normally like washing clothes all these things I will send to laundry and what else ah? ... Ok dressing, I dunno because I cannot see the colour ar. So I just simply err I take what I wear what loh. That's all only what. Oh I seldom buy clothes. I ... normally I ... the clothing leh normally I will get from maybe ah my relative ah, my uncle whoever give me the clothes ar.'

To be able to live independently suggests that S's disability does not make him a burden to his family. This is consistent with the Confucian values of filial piety, which are also very much linked to moral face. To have a child that not only is unable to care for his parents in their old age, but to still be a burden to them in adulthood can be regarded as a major loss of face, not only to the immediate family but including one's ancestors. Conservative Chinese society would regard a child like this as a punishment towards the entire family line for misdeeds in a past life. This is parallel with the discussions about *kamma* and disability in the *river* segment of this chapter and can also be the reason for stigma towards a family for having a disabled child – because of the assumption that the child would become a burden to parents in their old age. Hence, independent living can be regarded as an occupation of high VD, even more so for children born with disabilities. However, conservative Chinese families must first be able to recognise that independent living offers a possibility for them to get over the loss of face in the earlier stages and take the necessary action such children need.

Parent-Child / Elder-Younger relationships are among the key relationships outlined in Confucius' Five Cardinal Relationships (ruler-subject, spousal, and relationships between friends are also part of these). When these relationships are successfully conducted in line with the expectations outlined, conservative Chinese society regards them with approval. Reciprocity among these relationships is regarded as important. The elders are not solely at the giving end, there are also expectations for the young ones to give back, and this can be seen by S's mother making him 'do a lot of housework'. S does not necessarily see her demand as a bad thing, but regards it in a generally positive manner.

Based on S's descriptions, the elders of his family continue to show care to him even today as an adult (for example giving him clothes). However, it is interesting to note that S's narratives are primarily about how his elders have shown care to him while growing up and not about how he shows care to his elders. Perhaps his views on this matter would be something worth exploring further. They could be due to growing up in boarding school resulting in him becoming more Westernised and removed from conservative Chinese norms: in the *river* section of this chapter, he expresses anger towards his family's efforts at preserving the face of their larger self (by hiding him in a room away from visitors). His expectation that he should not be hidden away because 'we also human mar, they also human mar, right or not?' is more in line with Western values rather than Confucian ones.

Rocks: Obstacles to social inclusion among conservative Malaysian Chinese family members

> *'(BORN PREMATURE) Because other people, they scared you know. Like 2.5 pounds you imagine, 2.5 pounds how small is it? People, even my mother herself so, she want to take, she dare not also what ... Because they scared you know, because is very small you know. You see like the kitten like that you know. Very small you know ... I totally cannot see.'*

Fear, uncertainty and not knowing what to do, are commonly described by Malaysian parents when their children have birth defects or congenital disabilities. Approaches taken in response to this can differ from family to family, and is also dependent on the accessibility of disability services. S was very fortunate that his pragmatic grandmother made an effort to find out how to access those services so that he could engage in the VD occupations necessary for him to be able to regain face for the family, but this is not always the case for every family. As recently as 2010 when the first author spent some time on placement in the vocational training centre of the Malaysian Association for the Blind, she met a Malaysian Chinese lady in her early 30s who related that she had spent all her life kept at home. It was her first time experiencing formal education away from her family. This lady came from a rural area and thus very possibly from the sort of conservative Malaysian Chinese family described throughout this chapter. Further exploration from the perspective of these families would be helpful.

Conclusion: Using what we have learnt to 'create spaces'

Overall, it can be concluded that the *river flow* of S and his family pertaining specifically to his blindness has been significantly smooth, despite his complaints of feeling excluded in his younger days. S's intrinsic motivation in choosing to engage with occupations that happen to be in line with the VD expectations of conservative Chinese society has played an important part in enhancing his social inclusion at the family level, and probably the social inclusion of his family at the societal level as well.

As we can see from this chapter, face is the primary determinant of social inclusion in a conservative Chinese society. Therefore it is important to consider face and its implications for family and society when conducting intervention for BVI people coming from such families. The awareness of how occupations are connected to VD goals, HD goals and face can help occupational therapists facilitate their interventions better in line with the expectations of conservative Chinese families.

As conservative thinking families not only exist within the Malaysian Chinese community but also in other Malaysian cultures, it would be worth exploring whether the lessons learnt in this chapter could be adapted to their context as well. Cochrane and Gunderson (2012, p.33) introduce the idea of 'religious health assets' to promote better reception of health services among African communities. A similar approach in line with our local cultures could also be explored - mobilising 'cultural health assets' to promote culturally relevant approaches in support and education of Malaysian BVI people and their families.

What we have learnt about the relationship between occupation and social inclusion from this chapter could be helpful not only for occupational therapy practitioners in Malaysia in terms of developing culturally relevant approaches in their work, but also for practitioners in contexts working with not just pre-dominantly Chinese clients (Singapore, Taiwan, mainland China, Hong Kong) but also other Asian populations who have worldviews closer to Eastern / Chinese ones rather than the Western ones that stem from occupational therapy theory originating from North American. With globalisation and increasing human mobility, further exploration along the lines of what has been discussed in this chapter is necessary for occupational therapists around the world.

References

Carstens S. A. (2005) *Histories, cultures, identities: studies in Malaysian Chinese worlds.* Singapore: Singapore University Press

Central Intelligence Agency (2015) *The World Factbook.* [Accessed 16 September 2015 at https://www.cia.gov/library/publications/the-world-factbook/geos/my.html]

Cheng K.M. and Wong, K. C. (1996) School effectiveness in East Asia: Concepts, origins and implications. *Journal of Educational Administration,* 34, 5, 32-49

Chu, R. L. (1991) The threat to face and coping behavior. *Proceedings of the National Science Council.* Republic of China:Humanities and Social Science, 1, 14-31

Cochrane, J. R. and Gunderson, G. R. (2012) *The Barefoot Guide: Mobilising religious health assets for transformation.* [Accessed 12 September 2015 at www.barefootguide.org]

DeBernardi, J. (2004) *Rites of belonging: memory, modernity, and identity in a Malaysian Chinese community.* Stanford, CA: Stanford University Press

Department of Statistics Malaysia. (2010) *Population and Housing Census of Malaysia 2010.* Kuala Lumpur: Department of Statistics

Denison J. and Ooi, G. (1994) Disabled Peoples Movement in Malaysia. *Disability & Society.* 9, 1, 97-100

Goh, J. P. (2012) *'Chineseness' In Malaysian Chinese Education Discourse: The case of Chung Ling High School.* Masters thesis, University of Oregon

Han H. H. (2013) Taiwanese parents' reactions to the achievement of their children: Vertical distinctiveness versus horizontal distinctiveness. *The Asian Conference on Psychology & the Behavioral Sciences Official Conference Proceedings.* [Accessed 27 September 2015 at http://iafor.org/archives/offprints/acp2013-offprints/ACP2013_0128.pdf]

Ho, D. Y. F. (1976) On the concept of face. *American Journal of Sociology,* 81, 867-884

Hwang, K. K. and Han, K. H. (2010) Face and morality in Confucian society. *Oxford Handbook of Chinese Psychology.* New York: Oxford University Press

Hwang, K.K. (2012) Life goals and achievement motivation in Confucian society - foundations of Chinese psychology. *International and Cultural Psychology,* 1, 219-264

Iwama, M. K. (2006) *The Kawa Model; Culturally relevant occupational therapy.* Edinburgh: Churchill Livingstone-Elsevier Press

Lee, H. G. (2000) *Ethnic Relations In Peninsular Malaysia: The cultural and economic dimensions.* Singapore: Institute of Southeast Asian Studies

Lee, S. K. (2003) Exploring the relationship between language, culture and identity. *GEMA*

Online Journal of Language Studies, 3, 2, 1-13

Lee S. K. (2005) What price English? Identity constructions and identity in the acquisition of English. in S.K. Lee, S.M. Thang, and K. A. Baker (Eds.) *Language and Nationhood: New contexts, new realities.* SOLLS UKM: Bangi

Lee, K. H., and Tan, C. B. (Eds.). (2000) *The Chinese in Malaysia.* New York: Oxford University Press

Liang, C. J., Bedford, O. and Hwang, K. K. (2007). *Face due to the performance of a related other in a Confucian society.* Working paper for In Search of Excellence for the Chinese Indigenous Psychological Research Project, Department of Psychology, National Taiwan University

Nordin, M. (2001) Developing special education in each country and enhancing international mutualcooperation among countries in the Asia-Pacific Region (Malaysia).*22nd Asian and Pacific International Seminar on Special Education.* [Accessed 18 September 2015 at http://www.nise.go.jp/kenshuka/josa/kankobutsu/pub_d/d-175/d-175_1_6.pdf]

Reddy, S. C. and Tan, B.C. (2001) Causes of childhood blindness in Malaysia: Results from a national study of blind school students. *International Ophthalmology* 24,1, 53-59

Tan, L. E. (1997) The politics of Chinese education in Malaya, 1945-1961. *South-East Asian Historical Monographs.* Kuala Lumpur: Oxford University Press

Tan, T. J., Ho, W. F. and Tan, J. L. (2005) *The Chinese Malaysian contribution.* Kuala Lumpur: Centre for Malaysian Chinese Studies

Teoh, J. Y. (2011) *Lived experiences of Malaysian adults with visual impairments: A comparison between the Kawa Model and the Canadian Model of Occupational Performance.* Bachelors Honours thesis, Universiti Kebangsaan Malaysia

Wang, Q. and Chang L. (2010) Parenting and child socialization in contemporary China. *Oxford Handbook of Chinese Psychology.* New York: Oxford University Press

West, B. A. (2009) *Encyclopaedia of the Peoples of Asia and Oceania.* New York: Facts On File. p. 657

Wong, K. F., Lee K. S., Lee, S. K. and Azizah, Y. (2012) English use as an identity marker among Malaysian undergraduates. *The Southeast Asian Journal of English Language Studies*, 18, 1, 145 – 155

Chapter 4
Exclusion to inclusion of people with learning disabilities

Rhona Murray

Introduction

The treatment of many people with learning disabilities in the United Kingdom (UK) has been for centuries littered with cruelty, criminality and immorality. In recent decades however the majority of people with a learning disability have been empowered to achieve their aspirations through a combination of awareness raising, legislation and the development in the provision of support models that enable choices about where they live, who they live with, building relationships and access to education and occupation. There is no room for complacency as there continues to be overt discrimination and intolerable service provision. An example in Bristol, England, is Winterbourne View (Department of Health, 2012), a private hospital, where serious abuse of people with learning disabilities was exposed by an undercover BBC investigation. Subsequently there was a review of National Health Service (NHS) funded hospital placements, which can only be described as institutional care, for 3,400 people with learning disabilities.

Within living memory the exclusion of people with a learning disability was comprehensive. They were, in most instances, placed in large scale institutions, sometimes described as a 'hospital' that was usually on the outskirts of a town or a city. Their personal and social norms were inevitably skewed by staff, other patients and the environment of these institutions.

The concept of occupation was beginning to take root in the 1960s in institutions for people with learning disabilities, albeit the available occupation was defined by the limitations of the environment – buildings, other patients and staff. As people moved out of institutions, occupation opportunities gradually became available. Initially supported employment predominated but provision gradually opened up to mainstream opportunities in a variety of different sectors including retail, creative arts, hospitality, office work and supporting others.

Inclusion and occupation for people with learning disabilities demands the continual review of all practice, ensuring that the aspirations of people with a learning disability is delivered through safeguarding the potentially limitless scale and scope of inclusion and occupation. This approach is at the heart of all of the service provision.

The life experiences of two people who experienced family living, institutional care and are now living in their own home with support are included in this chapter. These case studies illustrate their personal development and the development of the services they received. Their exclusion, inclusion and occupation experiences are mirrored by many people with learning disabilities.

Defining learning disability

Learning disability is a phrase that has been applied to a wide range of people with a diversity of needs and abilities.

The British Institute of Learning Disabilities (BILD, 2011) provide three criteria that must be met before a learning disability can be diagnosed:

- intellectual impairment below an IQ score of 70;
- social or adaptive dysfunction combined with low IQ;
- early onset or later acquisition through injury of impairment.

In 2014, there were 26,786 adults with learning disability known to local authorities across Scotland. This equates to six people with learning disabilities per one thousand people in the general population (SCLID, 2015).

The evolution of understanding learning disability

The UK history of people with a learning disability provides an insight into mistreatment and exclusion from society. In the 19th Century the first legislation that was introduced that related to learning disability was the Lunacy Act 1845 and the Idiots Act 1886. In response to these Acts the Charity of the Asylum of Idiots was created in 1848. An example of the work in response to these Acts was the building of a number of asylums for people with learning disabilities and mental health issues. The development of an asylum near Reigate is described in a London Heritage Blog (Ianvisits, 2010) sourced from the *Illustrated London News* (March, 1854):

> The building will accommodate 400 inmates, classified in the following manner – 84 adult females; 66 adult males; 133 boys; 67 girls, 100 infants. The apartments will …. throughout be finished in a neat and pleasing, but at the same time economic, style.

This gives a sense that approaches to people with learning disabilities were beginning to change from the beginning of the 19th Century, when around 300 people were accommodated in nine charitable asylums.

In the first decade of the 20th Century Francis Galton founded the Eugenics Society. Eugenics became increasingly used throughout the first half of the 20th Century in the UK and America. It focused on sterilisation of people who were thought of as genetically inferior which were perceived by some as a health risk to society. Koch (2012) describes how similar principles are coming back in a new guise as bioethics. An interesting current bioethical dilemma relating to learning disabilities is the availability of a Downs Syndrome test for pregnant women in the UK to enable the decision of whether to abort. The test was recently improved upon to minimise the risk to the pregnant woman (Boseley, 2016). This is at extraordinary odds with the ethical and societal development of the inclusion of people with learning disabilities.

1908 saw the publication of *Mental Deficiency* by Tredgold, which was the reference text for health professionals for the next 50 years. It perpetuated a sense that the social problems stemmed from people with learning disabilities and mental health issues. Jones (1960, p. 60) commented on the longevity of the book, 'Time and experience were to modify views and a consideration of the revisions which Tredgold made in his book'. The Mental Deficiency Act 1913 introduced terms such as 'idiot', 'imbecile', 'feeble-minded' and 'moral imbecile'. It also enabled the institutionalisation of some women with illegitimate children, which continued in the UK until the early 1960s.

In the 1940s key legislation on education, disabled persons' employment, and the establishment of the National Health Service was introduced. Although these various Acts provided some progress there was still obvious exclusion and discrimination. For example in the Education Act (1944) people with learning disabilities were described as 'uneducable'. The 1950s and 1960s began to see changes in thinking in the direct provision of services, some rooted in civil liberty and others driven by cost. Health and education took some time to enable inclusion in their models of service. By the 1980s the closure of hospitals for people with learning disabilities was beginning to occur and group homes were seen as the primary alternative. The significance of the changes that were happening at that time is encapsulated by the three patients in Gogarburn Hospital (Edinburgh), who were members of the Patients' Committee in 1981, and won the right to vote in parliamentary elections (*Edinburgh Evening News*, 2014).

The NHS and Community Care Act 1990 accelerated the positive pace of change for people with a learning disability and contributed to a range of Acts being introduced that protected and enhanced rights. By the late 1990s the predominant care option for people with learning disabilities was discharge from the hospitals they were living in and moving to their own homes. The introduction of *The Same as You* (Scottish Executive, 2000), the Regulation of Care Act (2001) and the Adult Support and Protection Act (2007), started to shift the balance to the person with learning disabilities, supporting their choices and ensuring protection. The legal protection included safeguarding welfare, managing finances, regulation of services and staff, tighter compulsory measures of detention and the ability to self-direct their support.

All of these legislative changes signify the investment in the change of approach to people with learning disabilities. They enabled access to housing, trained and accountable staff, regulatory scrutiny of services and most crucially shifting support into being self-directed (Audit Scotland, 2014).

Case studies

The following case studies focus on the support of two people with learning disabilities who currently receive a service in a *core and cluster model*. The model was developed as an alternative to institutional and resettlement accommodation for people with a high dependency. The key principles are to enable a flexible service, deliver community integration and maximise independent living. The *core* is a building or property used as a staff base that will sometimes contain communal facilities and the *cluster* is a number of properties surrounding the core. The number of properties will depend on a variety of factors including:

- The size of the housing development;
- The capacity of the core;
- The level of needs of the people requiring support;
- Maintaining the principle of integration.
- A successful core and cluster model is based in a community that:
- Meets basic needs – shops, health and wellbeing services and transport;
- Has social, economic and cultural opportunities.

The people who volunteered for the case studies receive 24 hour services in their own homes. The very least they highlight is the fundamental changes in their accommodation and support. They also, albeit subjectively, provide a sense of the growth of the person to the point of making their own informed choices.

Case study 1

Kay has autism, a learning disability and dyspraxia; she lived with her parents and sisters until she was eight. She was then admitted to a hospital where she lived for three years before being moved to another hospital, Lennox Castle, which had the highest number of patients, 1,600, of any learning disability hospital in Scotland. She lived there for 32 years. She was sedated frequently to manage the challenging behaviours she displayed and was considered to be a danger to herself and others.

When the unit at the hospital closed, Kay was moved to a service providing care in the community and accommodation. She shared a house with seven other women. The main objective was to provide a safe environment for Kay and enable her to start to participate in activities in her local community, however Kay's behaviours made this difficult. They included running away, self-harming, pulling fixtures and fittings from walls, dismantling rooms, no awareness of personal safety, hiding belongings, stealing, touching strangers and other inappropriate behaviours in public places. Her placement was reviewed and she was then moved to a five person group home but with a higher ratio of staff but despite these positive improvements, similar behaviours were evident. Kay was then offered her own tenancy (she was able to consent to her tenancy agreement due to it being pictorial) with her own staff team to enable consistency in the support she received and implementation of routines. These routines were put in place to reduce the behaviours that Kay had been experiencing, due predominantly to over 40 years of institutionalisation. In all her previous accommodation she had to share with others with minimal privacy. She was now able to experience choice and, to some degree, privacy (she requires 24 hour support). The impact of one to one support, privacy and increased choice had a significant impact on her behaviour.

When Kay moved into her own tenancy she did continue to display challenging behaviour that sometimes formed patterns and cycles. A feature of her autism was she was self-focused and perceived the world around her only. She treated people as objects, and interacted mainly as a means of getting attention and had little appreciation of the impact on others.

A focus of her support was to ensure the maximisation of her ability to communicate and therefore extend her social inclusion. This included concentrating on her ability to communicate through improvement of her speech, gestures and signs, applications on an i-pad, talking / communication books, pictures and photographs. These tools have broadened her skill base and created multiple opportunities. For example, she has a permanent placement in music therapy, which in the past failed. Kay goes on regular holidays which she funds herself. These would have been very stressful for her in the past but are less so now due to her developed communication skills. Her attention and concentration span has increased. She now does not get angry when carrying out time consuming tasks.

She is fully involved in organising and controlling her support through a range of bespoke communication tools which has reduced repetitive behaviours. Examples include practical things such as times for meals, food choices or visiting friends and relatives. She has no choice however when she leaves her home, she has to be accompanied at all times due to the level of risk due to her capacity.

She is now able to reflect and communicate her past experiences in institutions and has explained how it made her feel angry and scared. She didn't like being forced to take medication and be given injections to sleep. She describes how she would pull out drips when she was given medication intravenously. She associates certain music with her experiences in hospital but can now hear it without reacting negatively because she says she feels safe and happy.

Case study 2

Ken lived with his parents up until the age of seven. He then moved to a service which provided residential care for children with learning disabilities. He had his own room but had to share other facilities.

Ken found it hard to conform to routine or behavioural expectations in a group environment and the consequences were that he became physically aggressive when he found a situation overwhelming. Ken moved into another service when he was 18, which was a large residential home with a mixture of male and female residents. He continued to exhibit aggression and also inappropriate sexualised behaviour with a female resident. The management of these incidents by staff resulted in him becoming anxious and withdrawn. He stayed in his bedroom for longer periods and eventually refused to come out at all, staying in bed all day and toileting in his bedroom.

The service was unable to break this cycle of self-neglect and Ken moved back home to live with his parents. After a few weeks he refused to leave his bedroom at his parents' house. He also became physically aggressive towards them which led to him being detained in hospital under the Mental Health Act. The priority at the hospital was to manage a specific behaviour, his tendency to withdraw and self-neglect. He made steady progress and as a consequence moved in with three other men with learning disabilities. After a few months Ken's mental health began to deteriorate and he began to follow old behaviour patterns of self-neglect.

He was referred to the challenging behaviour team (CBT), who initiated a programme of physical prompting in the mornings. The CBT managed this for a period of two weeks. This programme worked and enabled him to have a positive routine. Within a few days he had broken his old behaviour pattern and was able to enjoy his day activities.

He continued to live in a shared house for two more years. Ken then moved into his own flat. The move was initially successful and the staff were able to replicate his morning routine. Staff sought advice from the CBT about the positioning of the furniture in his bedroom, focusing on the environment and how it impacted him. It was the first time that he had his own environment and was able to make his own choices and he was supported to stay in touch with his former house mates and friends.

Ken moved again in 2009, with his own 24 hour all male team (the gender of team was defined due to repeated inappropriate infatuations with female staff members). This was an opportunity to once again review his support looking at the individual way that he experienced the world, how he understood things and how he communicated. At this time he was formally diagnosed with dyspraxia, a severe learning disability and autism. Initially the staff that supported him focused on how he likes to follow familiar routines and anticipates certain things in a sequence of events. They looked at his obsessive-compulsive tendencies which can make certain situations very stressful for him and provided him with ways to minimise the pressure he often felt when performing a task.

Ken makes his own decisions and does many things independently that he was unable to do previously. He is unable to communicate verbally, so the staff that work with him use sign-along and symbols to allow him space to communicate. By enabling him to express himself and supporting him to do things for himself, staff have assisted him in improving his self-esteem.

He now has a mobility car through a government funded mobility allowance. This makes going out less stressful for him because he has his own choice of space in the car. It addresses some of the sensory issues that he experiences that can make being out very confusing and stressful for him. He regularly stays with his family and he enjoys cars, pints of Guinness and photography.

Exclusion to inclusion

The case studies clearly highlight Kay and Ken's damaging early life experiences and in particular the transitions from living with family to institutional care, which inevitably guaranteed long term emotional trauma. This was then compounded by conditions and treatment that is likely to have closely mirrored what is repeatedly described in a range of reports on institutional care.

This generation's early days in institutional care, which particularly Kay experienced, is recognised by Morris (1969) who reported on 35 hospitals (90% of the learning disability population was in residential accommodation), noting that nothing had changed from a decade earlier when similar studies had been undertaken.

The style of support for Kay and Ken was stark. In most learning disability hospitals staff were trained to deal with negative behaviour through punishment and restraint which included the use of medication, isolation and physical restriction. There was no attempt to find out the cause. In most cases the choices of occupation would have been based on self-sufficiency, survival and boredom. The behaviour of many people when they moved from institutional care appeared to be a mixture of carried forward habitual behaviour as well as finding new ways of expression, which were not always in their best interests or those of the other people around them.

Ken and Kay's experiences reflect some of the fictional and factual accounts of people who experienced institutional care and life in their own homes and communities. David Cook's books *Walter* (1978) and *Winter Doves* (1979) and a BBC Radio 4 play *Walter Now* (2009) all track the milestones of someone with a learning disability without sentimentality, mirroring the very harsh social reality of community life for some people who had been liberated from institutional care.

A study by Hubert and Hollins (2006, p.7) on males with challenging behaviour who were being discharged from a locked hospital ward and provided with accommodation in the community exposed their experiences:

> The men's lives were emotionally, socially and physically deprived. Their individual, gender and social identities were not recognised, and their general health and mental health care needs were inadequately addressed.

There is not a lot of recent research to assess whether this continues to be the experience of people with learning disabilities. That could be due to the sense that the locked hospital wards are no longer prevalent. However in 2016 3,500 vulnerable people with learning disabilities are still resident in inpatient units. In an open letter to David Cameron, the UK Prime Minister at that time, the relatives of people in institutional care expressed their anger about the lack of urgency to move people with learning disabilities from inappropriate institutions (*Learning Disability Today*, 2016).

Removing barriers

Both Kay and Ken were guided and managed through the transition from institutional care to the maximisation of independent living. Establishing emotional and physical safety in their own home and then making connections with their chosen communities began the process of finding themselves and therefore increasing their independence.

Deinstitutionalisation is a long process and it is only in recent years that Kay and Ken are able to live their lives through having genuine choice and consequently being included in all of their chosen activities. Inclusion also requires access and there are a range of obstructions which are not exclusive to people with learning disabilities that can easily prevent connection with the community. Ensuring housing and amenities are designed in a way that provides for practical as well as health and wellbeing needs is crucial. Delivering meaningful social interaction and community connectedness with, if possible, the people that will be living there, is at the centre of influence of any design decisions.

People with profound learning disabilities require a barrier free environment i.e. no accessibility issues in their internal and external living spaces. Approaches which only rely on aids and adaptations are not the solution. Sadly there are few housing developments that could deliver barrier free housing due to the financial restraints of building bespoke housing; therefore the ability to freely access a life outside of their home is a significant restraint to the inclusion of people with profound learning disabilities. Exclusion still exists in their daily activities because of the unintentional physical restraint in some accommodation.

Kay and Ken both live in the same community with 24 hours resources. They have several communities aside from their neighbourhood and the wider community, in an area in Edinburgh, Scotland, where they are both actively involved. A recent example is their involvement in a time-banking scheme including its development and giving of their time. Volunteer Now (2016, p1/1) provide a definition of a time-bank:

'In a time-bank you earn time credits by giving practical help and support to others. One hour of service given earns you one credit. You can then exchange that credit for an hour of something that you need. In each case, everyone's time is equal.'

Negative occupation has been highlighted in previous pages. The definition of and the aspiration of occupation is provided by the World Federation of Occupational Therapy (2010, p1/1) and refers to

the everyday activities that people do as individuals, in families and with communities to occupy time and bring meaning and purpose to life. Occupations include things people need to, want to and are expected to do.

Choices of positive occupation for both Kay and Ken were severely limited in the institutions they lived in. They developed self-occupations that were driven by the physical and emotional restraint they experienced. It took some time to deinstitutionalise their restrained mode of occupation into genuine choice with the by-product of social inclusion, income, skills development, improved health and increased housing options. For example their occupation is focused on areas that mirror their interests and skills. Kay regularly attends Drake Music Scotland who describe their role as

making Scotland a place where ground-breaking new music featuring skilled musicians and composers with disabilities comes alive for everyone. (Drake Music Scotland, 2016)

The development of support must consider that choice is not stifled by accepting the easy social options (Forrester-Jones et al, 2006). For example the person being supported can view the person providing the service as part of their social option rather than the relationship merely being the conduit to social inclusion. If someone is to be socially included, the starting point is the inclusion must be authentic rather than contrived.

History repeating itself

The recent preventable death of Stephen Armstrong in hospital who had learning and physical disabilities, suggests that there was 'indirect discrimination' (Learning Disability Scotland, 2015, p.2) by health professionals. Michael Matheson, former Minister for Public Health, in his introduction in *The Keys of Life* (Scottish Government, 2013, p.4-5) stated,

to be truly accepted in society means being treated equally and fairly in other ways. It means having a health service that recognises and redresses the stark fact that people with learning disabilities still die 20 years earlier than the general population.

Exclusion and lack of occupation was clearly the experience for most people with learning disabilities before 1990. It is only in the past 25 years that there has been a sea change in attitudes rooted in the progress of civil rights, backed by legislation, towards the rights of people generally, but also specifically for people with learning disabilities many of whom have at the forefront of agitating for these changes.

However there can be no complacency. Following on from Winterbourne View, Mencap and The Challenging Behaviour Foundation published *Out of Sight* (2012) which highlighted 260 cases of neglect and abuse in institutional style provision. Jon Rouse, Director General for Social Care, Local Government and Care Partnerships stated

> Yes, some of these larger institutions have got to close. They are completely inappropriate in terms of modern-day care models. (Brindle, 2015)

Conclusion

It is evident that most people with learning disabilities now have the opportunity to live their lives based on their choices and aspirations but there is a sense that they are only less excluded rather than included, although it is undeniable their rights are far more significant in the 21st Century in Scotland in comparison to 50 years ago.

One of the significant and current threats to that progress in inclusion is reduction in funding. The provision of consistent, quality support cannot be achieved if the political agenda is solely cost reduction. The introduction of outcome based payments (CCPS et al, 2010) for the provision of support appears as if it may be of value to all stakeholders because it has the potential to provide creative, life enhancing choice. If the current strategy to funding remains, there is an inevitability that people with learning disabilities will begin to lose the momentum of positive change that ensures occupation, social inclusion, choice and their independence.

Despite these challenges the self-empowerment of people with learning disabilities will ensure they will take the lead in challenging and demanding their rights to support that provides their aspirations.

This poem in *The Keys to Life* (Scottish Government, 2013) was written by a group of service users from South Lanarkshire. It neatly encompasses the mind-set for that to happen.

Ten Years ago, The Same as You?
Raised people's awareness of what to do
To stop separation and isolation and encourage social integration
And now finally people listen to what we say
We're onwards and upwards – we're here to stay.

References

Adult Support and Protection (Scotland) Act 2007 [Accessed 13 July 2016 at http://www.legislation.gov.uk/asp/2007/10/contents]

Learning Disability Alliance Scotland (2015) Remembering Stephan Armstrong. in *Alliance News, 53, p2*. [Accessed 26 September 2015 at http://www.ldascotland.org/docs/Newsletter%20august%202015.pdf]

Audit Scotland (June 2014) *Self Directed Support, Audit Commission and Auditor General.* [Accessed 4 October 2015 at http://www.audit-scotland.gov.uk/docs/central/2014/nr_140612_self_directed_support.pdf]

Boseley, S. (2016) NHS to offer safer Down's syndrome test to pregnant women. *The Guardian.* [Accessed 7 September 2015 at https://www.theguardian.com/society/2016/oct/29/safer-downs-syndrome-test-nhs-pregnant-women-nipt]

Brindle, D. (2015) Is the spectre of Winterbourne View finally beginning to shift? *The Guardian* (11 February) [Accessed on 2 June 2016 at http://www.theguardian.com/social-care-network/2015/feb/11/winterbourne-view-learning-disability-nhs]

The British Institute of Learning Disabilities (BILD) (2011) *Fact sheet: Learning Disabilities.* [Accessed 10 October 2015 at http://www.bild.org.uk/information/factsheets/]

Community Care Providers (CCPS), Housing Support Enabling Unit (HSEU) and Voluntary Sector Social Services Workforce Unit (VVSSWU) (2010) *An outcomes approach in social care and support: an overview of current frameworks and tools.* [Accessed 13 July 2016 at http://www.ccpscotland.org/wp-content/uploads/2014/01/outcomes-briefing.pdf]

Cook, D. (1978) *Walter.* Harmondsworth: Penguin.

Cook, D. (1979) *Winter Doves.* Harmondsworth: Penguin.

Cook, D. (2009) *Walter Now.* [BBC Radio 4 play]. [Accessed 8 June 2016 at https://www.amazon.co.uk/Walter-Now-BBC-Radio-Saturday/dp/B004SHIXZK]

Department of Health (2012) *Transforming Care: A national response to Winterbourne View Hospital. Department of Health Review: Final Report* [Accessed 4 October at https://www.gov.uk/government/uploads/system/uploads/attachment_data/file/213215/final-report.pdf]

Drake Music Scotland [Accessed 2 June 2016 at http://drakemusicscotland.org]

Edinburgh Evening News (2014) Obituary Jimmy McIntosh MBE 5th June 2014 [Accessed 2 June 2016 at http://www.edinburghnews.scotsman.com/news/obituary-jimmy-mcintosh-mbe-74-1-3434026]

Forrester-Jones, R., Carpenter, J., Coolen-Schrijner, P., Cambridge, P., Tate, A., Beecham, J., Hallam, A., Knapp, M. and Wooff, D. (2006) The social networks of people with learning disabilities living in the community twelve years after resettlement from long-stay hospitals. *Journal of Applied Research in Intellectual Disabilities*, 19, 285-295

HM Government (1944) Education Act (1944). [Accessed 4 October 2015 at http://www.legislation.gov.uk/ukpga/Geo6/7-8/31/contents/enacted]

Hubert, J. and Hollins, S. (2006) Men with severe learning disabilities and challenging behaviour in long-stay hospital care – Qualitative study. *British Journal of Psychiatry*,188, 1, 70-74

Ianvisits (2010) *A New Asylum for Idiots.* [sourced from The Illustrated London News, March 1854. Accessed 13 July 2016 at https://www.ianvisits.co.uk/blog/2010/05/12/a-new-asylum-for-idiots/]

Jones, K. (1960) *Mental Health and Social Policy, 1845-1959.* London: Routledge

Koch, T. (2012) *Thieves of Virtue. How bioethics stole the world*. Cambridge, Mass: MIT Press.

Learning Disability Today (2016) *Families of people abused at Winterbourne View call for urgent action to help people with learning disabilities.* [Accessed 7 September 2015 at https://www.learningdisabilitytoday.co.uk/families-of-people-abused-at-winterbourne-view-call-for-urgent-action-to-help-people-with-learning-disabilities]

Mencap and The Challenging Behaviour Foundation (2012) *Out of Sight: Stopping the neglect and abuse of people with a learning disabilities.* [Accessed 15 September 2015 at https://www.mencap.org.uk/sites/default/files/2016-08/Out-of-Sight-Report.pdf]

Mental Deficiency Act (1913). [Accessed 4 October 2015 at http://www.ncbi.nlm.nih.gov/pmc/articles/PMC2987037/]

Morris, P. (1969) *Put Away: A sociological study of institutions for the mentally retarded.* London: Routledge & Kegan Paul

NHS and Community Care Act (1990) [Accessed 2 June 2016 at http://www.legislation.gov.uk/ukpga/1990/19/contents]

Regulation of Care (Scotland) Act (2001) (UK Government). [Accessed 2 June 2016 at http://www.legislation.gov.uk/asp/2001/8/contents]

Scottish Executive (2000) *The Same as You? A review of services for people with learning disabilities.* [Accessed 4 October 2015 at http://www.gov.scot/resource/doc/1095/0001661.pdf]

Scottish Government (2013) *Keys to Life: Improving quality of life for people with learning disabilities.* Edinburgh: Scottish Government [Accessed 15 September 2015 at http://www.gov.scot/resource/0042/00424389.pdf]

Scottish Consortium for Learning Disabilities (SCLID) (2015) *Learning Disability Statistics Scotland, 2014.* A National Statistics Publication for Scotland 2015. [Accessed 15 October 2015 http://www.scld.org.uk/wp-content/uploads/2015/08/Learning-Disability-Statistics-Scotland-2014-report.pdf]

Tredgold, A.F. (1908) *Mental Deficiency (Amentia).* New York: William Wood and Co.

Volunteer Now (2016) *Timebanking.* [Accessed on 2 June 2016 http://www.volunteernow.co.uk/volunteering/timebanking]

The World Federation of Occupational Therapists (2010) *Definition of Occupational Therapy.* [Accessed on 2 June 2016 at http://www.wfot.org/aboutus/aboutoccupationaltherapy/definitionofoccupationaltherapy.aspx]

Chapter 5
Promoting occupation-based social inclusion: Scanning the legislative environment in Zimbabwe

Tecla Mlambo, Nyaradzai Munambah,
Clement Nhunzvi, Fambaineni Innocent Magweva,
and Tatenda John Maphosa

Introduction

The importance of occupation in human life as well as the importance of enabling factors for inclusiveness, access and equal opportunities cannot be overemphasised. Disability, chronic illness, poverty, lack of opportunity and access can hinder someone from participating in health promoting occupations. Multiple aspects are important when one thinks of enabling occupations, and these can be individual or societal. Both individual and societal factors are influenced by the legislative and policy environment as well as the culture and values of the people. Inclusion of persons with disabilities in everyday activities involves encouraging them to have roles similar to their non disabled peers, and it also requires making sure that adequate policies and practices are in place.

The legislative and policy contexts are therefore crucial as far as facilitation of access to basic needs, health, rehabilitation, education and work are concerned. According to the Free Dictionary (www.thefreedictionary.com/policy), a policy is defined as

> a plan of or course of action, as of a government, political party, or business, and is intended to influence and determine decisions, actions, and other matters.

Legislation is a law or set of laws enacted by a government or international body. Policies are usually derived from the legislation.

This chapter will discuss the legislative framework in Zimbabwe as regards equal opportunities for occupation and support for social inclusion. As we believe change in occupational therapy practice is important in Zimbabwe, we end by proposing a framework for occupation-based social inclusion which occupational therapists and related rehabilitation professionals can use.

Occupation and social inclusion

The term social inclusion is difficult to define, however, it is linked to equal opportunities for participation (Davys & Tickle, 2008). Individuals denied opportunities for meaningful participation in the community become socially excluded because of a number of factors that include stigma, dislocation from networks, illness, poverty, and barriers such as inaccessible transport, finances and distance to services (Russell & Lloyd, 2004). Often these people are denied opportunities and cannot access advocates of equalisation of opportunities. In addition, they often cannot obtain the resources they require to engage and participate in meaningful occupations in the community. This leads to occupational injustice, which is the limited exposure to opportunities and choice resulting in limited development of one's potential (Townsend & Wilcock, 2004).

Enabling participation is often espoused as a strategy to promote inclusion, social justice and equality (Gannon & Nolan, 2007). Therefore, disability should be approached through a human rights perspective, advocating for equalisation of opportunities. The 'doings' of individuals or groups in society are a vehicle through which participation and ultimately inclusion can be achieved (Whiteford & Pereira, 2012). This is also highlighted by Wilcock (2006) who noted that the process of doing, being, becoming and belonging through occupations is essential in promoting health, wellbeing and social inclusion in various cultural, economic, institutional, social and political contexts.

For the social inclusion of the excluded, there is need to address the barriers to occupational participation in all areas of life, including education, employment, leisure, self-care and citizenship, with the goal of empowering all people involved to have an equal chance for participation in society (Samyshkin et al, 2010).

Occupation has a transformative potential on an individual's health if the individual can choose and engage in meaningful occupations for the purposes of realising one's dreams (Kuo, 2011). Moreover, the value and meaning derived from participation in an occupation does not only benefit the individual, but the communities where they live, work and play (Leclair, 2010). In addition, occupation influences the society by providing the mechanism for social interaction, social development and growth, thereby forming the foundation of community, local and national identity (Wilcock, 2006). Thus, occupation has both a cultural and economic influence, or rather an interdependence of many factors (Whiteford & Pereira, 2012), and this is linked to geo-political factors such as the local environment and the possibilities this affords (Leclair, 2010; Wilcock, 2006).

International and national legislation to support occupation-based social inclusion

With occupation being a basic human right and need, Wilcock (2006) proposed that an occupational perspective on public health (including social inclusion) be adopted in which population health needs are met by addressing the occupational needs and occupational risks of the individual, the group and the community. Occupation-based social inclusion is important for marginalised groups whose human rights are usually infringed on.

An overarching social inclusionary factor is legislation. Without strategies and resources for the implementation of legislation and policies, occupation-based social inclusion remains a dream even in a context with sound legislature. Several exclusionary factors may exist and may need to be addressed, and these include but are not limited to low or lack of income, poverty, unemployment, lack of access to credit facilities, crime, lack of safety, unavailability of services and facilities, disunity in the community, disability, disempowerment, restricted choices, lack of access to information, lack of representation, isolation, low education levels and insufficient time for participation (Kenyon, 2003). However, not all the above exclusionary factors can be addressed by legislation and policy alone. Isolation, disunity in the community and lack of safety for example, would require processes to do with culture, values and beliefs other than legislative. These may require a cultural transformation enacted at an interpersonal level, which is beyond the scope of this chapter. The implementation of legislature and policies can be affected by an unstable economic and political environment.

For a successful implementation of occupation-based social inclusion, there is need for an appreciation of the legislation and policies at both international and national levels. Treaties and conventions are considered international law whose relevance to a country depend on whether a country is a signatory to the aforementioned or not (United Nations, 2015). By signing a convention/treaty, a country agrees to be bound by such international law and is expected to introduce appropriate laws and policies to implement or operationalise the convention statutes. By ratifying or signing a convention, a state commits to ensuring that national law will guarantee rights enumerated in that convention (Pal et al, 2010).

Zimbabwe is a signatory to several conventions/treaties that support occupation based social inclusion. Examples of such instruments are the United Nations Convention on the Rights of Children (UNCRC) (United Nations, 1989) and the United Nations Convention on the Rights of Persons with Disabilities (UNCRPD) (United Nations, 2006). The UNCRPD is the major document that informed the current Zimbabwean Constitution (Parliament of Zimbabwe, 2013) in terms of inclusion of persons with disabilities. Articles 1, 3, 5 – 7, 9, 10, 13, 19, 21, 24 -30 of the UNCRPD speak to issues of inclusion (United Nations, 2006) and the same issues are addressed in some way by the Zimbabwean Constitution (Parliament of Zimbabwe, 2013).

Declarations are also international instruments which are not always legally binding. Parties declare certain aspirations, although they can be regarded as treaties in the generic sense when intended to be binding at international law (United Nations, 2015). It is therefore important to establish whether there was an intention by parties to create binding obligations or not. Some declarations which originally were not intended to have binding force may gain that force with time based on their perceived relevance to an important cause, such as the 1948 Universal Declaration of Human Rights (United Nations, 2015). Zimbabwe is a signatory to the Universal Declaration of Human rights.

There are also guidelines and declarations at global or regional levels like the World Health Organization (WHO) guidelines on various health issues including Community Based Rehabilitation (CBR) (WHO, ILO, & IDDC UNESCO, 2010). These provide a framework for countries to use in addressing an issue and may be regarded as international policy. Zimbabwe, being a member of the World Health Organization and the United Nations is usually guided by such documents.

However, the real process of internationalisation usually takes place at the institutional or national level which has an important influence on the international dimension through policy, funding, programmes, and regulatory frameworks (Knight, 2004). As far back as the 1970s, it was however noted that there was an implicit assumption in most policy studies that once a policy has been formulated, the policy will be implemented (Smith, 1973). Smith (1973) noted that the assumption was invalid for policies formulated in many developing nations, where governments tended to formulate broad, sweeping policies, and where there were governmental bureaucracies which often lacked the capacity for implementation. Lack of resources to implement policies on empowerment and inclusion is a major issue in resource limited settings (Munemo & Tom, 2013; Levers et al, 2010). There is therefore need for interest groups and affected individuals and groups to influence the implementation of policy, which they often do (Smith, 1973).

Social inclusion in the context of Zimbabwean legislation

Countries' constitutions are the supreme laws of nations which form the basis for other national laws and policies. Where the law and constitutional provisions do not agree, the constitution reigns supreme, and Zimbabwe is no exception as the new constitution reiterates the same (Parliament of Zimbabwe, 2013).

We propose that one should look for certain words/terms and phrases in these legislative documents when investigating whether a country has a legislative framework in place for social inclusion or not. These are terms that can show support for social inclusion, such as: human rights and freedoms, inherent dignity and worth, equality and non-discrimination, equitable development, empowerment, affirmative action, achievement of full potential, access, equal opportunities, non-segregation, non-marginalisation, participation in community and family, employment and recreational activities, among others. These words and many more attest to social inclusion and are part of the Zimbabwean Constitution (Parliament of Zimbabwe, 2013).

Although the Constitution of Zimbabwe protects all people, there are specific groups that are singled out. These are considered vulnerable groups and are; children, women, youth, elderly persons, persons with disabilities and veterans of the liberation struggle (Parliament of Zimbabwe, 2013). In section 13 dealing with national development, the state and all institutions and agencies are encouraged to 'protect and enhance the right to equal opportunities in development' (Parliament of Zimbabwe, 2013, p19). In the next section on empowerment and employment creation, they are also 'to facilitate and take measures to empower through appropriate, transparent, fair and just affirmative action all marginalised persons, groups and communities in Zimbabwe'. When it comes to children and youth (Parliament of Zimbabwe, 2013), sections 19 and 20 stress access to appropriate education and training. In addition, reasonable measures must be taken to ensure that the youth are given opportunities to be represented and participate in political, social, economic and other spheres of life. There is also a mention of opportunities for recreational activities and access to relevant facilities for the youth. Similarly, regarding the elderly, section 21 calls for the facilitation of their participation in the life of their communities and for them to be given opportunities to engage in productive activities suited to their abilities (Parliament of Zimbabwe, 2013). All the above is clear evidence of social inclusion being addressed in the national legislation.

Section 22 (Parliament of Zimbabwe, 2013), in addition to other generic rights, states that persons with disabilities should be assisted in achieving their full potential and minimise the disadvantages they experience. There should also be work programmes consistent with their capabilities which are acceptable to them. Their special requirements must be considered and prioritised in development plans, and buildings and amenities must be accessible to them. In Section 23 on veterans (Parliament of Zimbabwe, 2013), economic empowerment is the main focus. Subsection 1 of section 24 on work and labour relations urges the state and its institutions and agencies to adopt policies and measures to 'provide everyone with an opportunity to work in a freely chosen activity, in order to secure a decent living for themselves and their families' (Parliament of Zimbabwe, 2013, p. 22). Subsection 2 further urges the same to secure

(a) full employment;
(b) the removal of restrictions that unnecessarily inhibit or prevent people from working and otherwise engaging in gainful economic activities;
(c) vocational guidance and the development of vocational and training programmes, including those for persons with disabilities; and
(d) the implementation of measures such as family care that enable women to enjoy a real opportunity to work.
(Parliament of Zimbabwe, 2013, p. 22).

Specific mention is made of equal opportunities in the education of the girl child in section 27, while the right to equal opportunities in political, economic, cultural and social spheres for men and women is mentioned in section 56 on equality and non-discrimination. In the same section 56, the constitution advocates for equality and non-discrimination of people with disabilities in various spheres of life including economic.

Section 83 of the Constitution of Zimbabwe (Parliament of Zimbabwe, 2013, p. 39) is again devoted to the rights of persons with disabilities where the state is urged to

take appropriate measures, within the limits of the resources available to it, to ensure that persons with disabilities realise their full mental and physical potential, including measures
a) to enable them to become self-reliant;
(b) to enable them to live with their families and participate in social, creative or recreational activities;
(c) to protect them from all forms of exploitation and abuse;

(d) to give them access to medical, psychological and functional treatment;

(e) to provide special facilities for their education; and

(f) to provide State-funded education and training where they need it.

All the above attest to constitutional support for occupation-based social inclusion, although professional groups and Disabled Persons Organisations (DPOs) are concerned about the recurrent phrase 'within the limits of the resources available to it' throughout the constitution. In addition to a constitution which strongly supports occupation-based social inclusion of marginalised groups, Zimbabwe also has several Acts of Parliament that support inclusion as shown in Table 1 (Parliament of Zimbabwe, 1972; 1985; 1987; 1992a; 1992b; 1995; 1996; 2008). There are many other legislative documents that support inclusion.

Table 1: Examples of Zimbabwean Acts of Parliament that support inclusion

Children's Act Chapter 5:06 of 1972
Labour Act of 1985
Education Act Chapter 25:04 of 1987
Disabled Persons Act Chapter 17:01 of 1992a
Land Acquisition Act Chapter 20:10 of 1992b
Public Health Act of 1995
War Veterans Act of 1995
Mental Health Act of 1996
Indigenization and Economic Empowerment Act of 2008

Of the Acts mentioned above, the Disabled Persons Act (Parliament of Zimbabwe, 1992a) directly speaks to inclusion of persons with disabilities. Among other things, the Disabled Persons Act provides for the appointment of a Director of Disabled Persons' affairs. This is a public service employee who is responsible for establishing the National Disability Board, and directing and coordinating the activities of institutions, associations and organisations concerned with the welfare and rehabilitation of persons with disabilities. The Board is mandated to formulate and develop measures and policies designed:

'(i) to achieve equal opportunities for disabled persons by ensuring, so far as possible, that they obtain education and employment, participate fully in sporting, recreation and cultural activities and are afforded full access to community and social services;

(ii) to enable disabled persons, so far as possible, to lead independent lives;

(iii) to give effect to any international treaty or agreement relating to the welfare or rehabilitation of disabled persons to which Zimbabwe is a party;

(iv) to prevent discrimination against disabled persons resulting from or arising out of their disability;

(v) to encourage and put into operation schemes and projects for the employment of or generation of income by disabled persons who are unable to secure employment elsewhere;

(vii) to encourage and secure the establishment of vocational rehabilitation centres, social employment centres and other institutions and services for the welfare and rehabilitation of disabled persons. (Parliament of Zimbabwe, 1992a, p. 2)

Zimbabwe's Constitution and several Acts of Parliament therefore support occupation-based social inclusion. What are required are clear policies that directly address disability and rehabilitation issues among others. Fowler (2000) highlighted the need to define the policy issue clearly if it has to be perceived as important. If a policy is not perceived as important by a large number of people, it will never attract enough attention to reach the policy agenda so that it may be considered to become formal policy (Fowler, 2000). A policy consistent with the Constitution and Acts of Parliament is more likely to get support from the important offices.

Good coverage of disability issues in the new Zimbabwean Constitution is a reflection of the active involvement of the Disability Board provided for by the Disabled Persons Act of 1992. Although the Board's operations have been affected by financial constraints, its voice is being heard by Government. Through active lobbying, people with disabilities managed to get two seats reserved in Parliament for a male and a female person with disabilities. Although the aim is a 10% quota for persons with a disability in Parliament, this is an encouraging starting point. It took the Disability Board more than 20 years to develop a National Disability Policy for Zimbabwe. At the time of writing, the policy document was awaiting Cabinet approval. It is also envisaged by the disability and rehabilitation fraternity in Zimbabwe that the Disabled Persons Act will be revised to reflect current legislation especially the current Constitution.

However, it is important to note that the efforts of all relevant stakeholders (the Disability Board, DPOs, Ministry of Health and Child Care, training institutions for Rehabilitation personnel such as the University of Zimbabwe, professional associations, professionals' regulatory authorities, academics, researchers etc) are not well coordinated, for what the disability activists term 'historical reasons' (Personal communication with Chairman of Disability Board). Disability and rehabilitation were introduced under different ministries with different ways of interpreting and utilising different disability models yet without a framework in place to link them. This has subsequently caused fragmented and uncoordinated service, hence, the evident need for harmonisation for greater impact. There is a tendency for stakeholders to take extreme viewpoints, such as being proponents of the social model of disability only at the expense of the medical and rehabilitation needs of certain categories or vice versa. However, there is a need to acknowledge and respect diversity within people with disabilities themselves, for example, people with hearing impairment often have very different perspectives to other people with disabilities because their disability is less immediately visible. Those with paraplegia secondary to spinal cord injury or disease, for example, may have more medical and rehabilitation needs than others. Schneider et al. (2012) also noted that grouping of people with diverse needs makes it difficult for effective policy implementation.

Occupation-based social inclusion from the Disabled People's Organisations' perspective

The information that follows is based on desk reviews and interviews with the

Secretariats for two major organisations that represent people with disabilities, the National Association of Societies for the Care of the Handicapped (NASCOH) and the Federation of Disabled People's Organisations of Zimbabwe (FODPZ).

NASCOH was founded in 1969 and represents 70 organisations that work with people with disabilities. These organisations represented by NASCOH can be categorised into three groups, namely service providers (rehabilitation centres and institutions caring for people with disabilities), professional bodies, and DPOs. NASCOH is therefore an umbrella body that represents issues to do with disability and rehabilitation in Zimbabwe. Its major roles are coordination of the member organisations, playing an advisory role to the government on disability issues, capacity building and programme implementation.

NASCOH effects its advisory role to the government through the Disability Board which is an arm of the government that was established by an Act of Parliament. Its members also sit in several inter-ministerial portfolio committees, such as, Psychomotor, Indigenisation and Empowerment, Information Communication Technology (ICT), Sports Council, Youth Council, Media Commission, Gender Commission, Tourism, Education etc. Their main purpose in these committees is to promote inclusion of people with disabilities in all sectors of society. NASCOH has been fighting for a Disability desk in each government ministry. In response to the call for recognition of the human rights of people with disabilities, NASCOH developed models and approaches to redressing the exclusion of persons with disabilities, focused on building structures at community, district, and provincial levels in order to fight disability discrimination at all levels. At the time of writing the structures were as depicted in Figure 1.

Figure 1: Structure of NASCOH in 2016

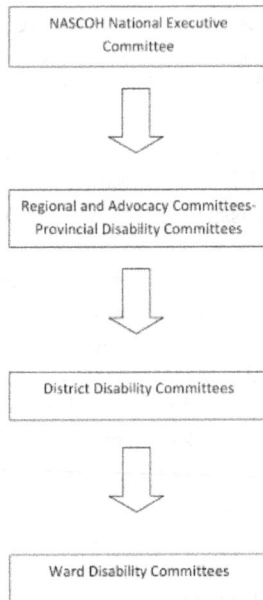

NASCOH National Executive Committee

↓

Regional and Advocacy Committees-Provincial Disability Committees

↓

District Disability Committees

↓

Ward Disability Committees

The Ward Disability Committees include people with disabilities and community leaders, such as councilors, chiefs, headmen and other influential people in the communities. All this is meant to promote inclusion of people with disability from grassroots levels. The chairperson of the Ward Disability Committee sits on the Ward Development Committee so that there is mainstreaming of disability issues in all development projects in the communities. The Ward Disability Committees (WDCs), a disability inclusion structure established by NASCOH and its member organisations at community level in 14 districts, are endowed with the skills and capacities for people with disabilities to take effective charge of their lives and to spearhead the mainstreaming of disability and their inclusion in all spheres of life. These innovative citizen engagement structures (ward disability committees) are tasked with ensuring access to economic, political, and social opportunities for persons with disabilities and enhancing the participation and inclusion of persons with disabilities in their respective wards.

FODPZ is an umbrella organisation for Disabled People's Organisations (Kupe & Mazula, 2010). It calls itself the legal voice for DPOs. It was formed in 2003 and its members are 12 national representative organisations of people with disability and parents of children with disabilities. Its main mandate is on policy and advocacy, while grassroots work is done by specific DPOs on the ground. It is important to note that FODPZ members are also members of NASCOH. FODPZ has not been very proactive due to the economic/political situation that has been prevailing in the country, which has been associated with donor fatigue. FODPZ, like NASCOH, is advocating for the national prioritisation and mainstreaming of disability issues, such as inclusion of sign language in all teacher training schools and primary schools, physical accessibility of the school environment to all, and more emphasis on psychomotor skills.

Both NASCOH and FODPZ admit that there are strategies in place to integrate people with disability but they need more in terms of resources and implementation. Their major success stories include their participation in the Constitution making process (leading to the comprehensive coverage of disability issues in the current Zimbabwean Constitution), being consulted in drafting the first report on the implementation of the UNCRPD in Zimbabwe and being given the opportunity to give their input on national issues through their participation in various inter-ministerial committees.

Despite these successes, there are still some gaps in implementation which stem from some loopholes in the same Constitution. Clauses such as 'within the limits of the resources available to it' do not compel the government to provide resources for implementation of constitutional rights. This is typical of government documentation in many cases. In an analysis of eleven African Union policy documents Schneider et al (2012) noted the broad nature and lack of detailed specifications of policy documents when it came to issues that affect vulnerable groups. As a result, implementation is slow or non-existent. A National Disability Policy was developed by DPOs through the Ministry of Public Service and Social Welfare, which is a parent ministry for disability issues, highlighting the importance of a policy that is government initiated, supported and implemented. However, it is taking too long for the government to adopt it, and their main excuse is lack of resources. This excuse is stemming from a vacuum in the Constitution in terms of the government's mandate to provide resources for implementation (Magweva et al., 2012). Although Zimbabwe was one of the first African countries to introduce a Disability Act and a Disability Board, it has been left behind by many countries in terms of implementation (Levers et al., 2010). The Disability Board is currently under the poorly resourced Ministry of Public Service and Social Welfare Directorate.

The appointment of Parliamentarians representing disability was a major achievement for the disability fraternity in Zimbabwe. Yet for the Parliamentarians to be effective there is the need to equip them and provide support to their offices for more effective representation of the persons with disabilities. The process of creating and maintaining a robust and effective community level disability structure, so that it is able to pick up on or to identify real issues, engage solution holders at community level and feed the Parliamentarians with issues to be tabled in parliament, is centred on the training of ward disabilities committees. These community level disability structures require continual renewal to maintain their value and effectiveness. Although this model of representation and the organisation underpinning it is considerable, there may still be problems of representing people with disabilities from within the disability movement. For example, there is the tendency for representation to go to people who are more articulate and vocal, discriminations operate within the disability network, that is, against those with invisible disabilities, cognitive and mental health problems (Armstrong, 2002). It is however heartening to note that in Zimbabwe, there are various disability specific groups that form the NASCOH as a way of ensuring comprehensive coverage of the issues that affect these different groups.

Furthermore, the Zimbabwean Ministry of primary and secondary education, rehabilitation professionals, people with disability and other disability activists are advocating for inclusive education. Implementation is still low due to lack of resources. Great challenges are being witnessed in the sector where only those with mild disabilities can be accommodated due to physical barriers (e.g. lack of ramps); there is no access to health and rehabilitation services in schools, no access to assistive devices and a shortage of adequately resourced teachers. The lack of rehabilitation services throughout the school system, starting in early childhood development (ECD), hinders early identification and intervention which are critical in preventing later exclusion (Levers et al, 2010). In addition, children with disabilities in schools are not given enough time to develop independent skills before they reach tertiary level. Teachers focus on academic skills forgetting that a child with disability may need to be trained in self-care, independent mobility and other skills. Special education teachers have not been trained to handle the various other needs of children with disabilities. Although that gap can be filled by rehabilitation personnel, there are other areas that need to be addressed such as the adaptation of examinations for those who use sign language. Many fail to get good grades in their final school examinations and become illegal street vendors instead of gaining formal employment (Levers et al, 2010). In terms of skills development, the Ministry of Youth has achieved the integration of most disability categories except persons with hearing impairment.

Positive strides have been made in the education and health sectors in terms of including people with disability in employment, however, a lot still needs to be done in other public as well as private sectors. With no legislation that compels someone to employ a quota of people with disability and no accompanying tax incentives, there is no obligation on companies to do so. There is minimum participation of people with disability in community development programmes, although the need to develop and strengthen grassroots structures is highlighted by more participation witnessed in those districts with structures in place.

In moving forward, DPOs are advocating for the amendment to the Constitution and Disabled Persons Act to make government and stakeholders fully responsible for the implementation of the inclusion agenda through mandatory provision of resources. Zimbabwe has been experiencing economic problems that have left several, if not all, government ministries underfunded. However, the available limited resources could be more equitably distributed to implement legislation to support inclusion of people with disabilities. This will guard against the major problem of non-implementation. Occupation-based social inclusion needs prioritisation by the government, donor communities and their implementing partners. Research is also necessary if evidence based social inclusion is to be promoted. Overall, self-advocacy from a united front like NASCOH by people with disabilities, service providers, professional bodies and DPOs is required.

Steps that occupational therapists can take to facilitate occupation-based social inclusion

This section explores where occupational therapy in Zimbabwe is at in relation to the legislative context and tries to provide proposals for moving forward towards social inclusion. Occupation-based interventions provide tools that can be used to promote social inclusion in a variety of contexts. Addressing or presenting issues from a legislative point of view puts people from different viewpoints on a level footing in terms of understanding the legal provisions and implications of not addressing certain issues.

Although occupational therapists have always known the importance of independence in self-care, work and leisure, they have not always been advocates of these for all populations. In Zimbabwe, occupational therapists are primarily aligned with the medical model (Personal experiences of authors), overlooking the fact that some of the sicknesses and injuries may be caused by social determinants, rather than individual medical concerns. This is shown by the rise in cases of mental illness and substance abuse among Zimbabweans since the nation started experiencing economic hardships, which are coupled with high unemployment rates and difficult life circumstances (Mlambo et al, 2014).

Professionals have an important role to play in facilitating inclusion as they often deal with the underlying causes of exclusion at both individual and societal levels. Professionals can also create boundaries and find themselves repressed, for example, just focusing on the medical model when they can extend their borders to include other models. As a result there may be infighting among related professionals to the detriment of the client, professions and national development. According to the 2014 Medical Rehabilitation Practitioners Council of Zimbabwe (MRPCZ) register, there were 128 registered occupational therapists, and of these 102 (79.7%) were employed in government hospitals (MRPCZ, 2014). Occupational therapists employed in government institutions in Zimbabwe are mainly working with acute cases in a hospital setting. This predominance is probably due to the way occupational therapy was introduced during the colonial era under the aegis of the medical establishment, making it difficult for occupational therapists to establish an occupational basis and professional autonomy for their work (Joubert, 2010). That left a medical legacy and thus restricting occupational therapy practice domains and scope, a predisposition that might lead to apathy. By working within a medical model, theoretical models used by most occupational therapists in Zimbabwe are aligned with treatment of the individual's illness or disease and therefore, may not take full account of social causes as well as not relating well to the local context (Joubert, 2010).

Another explanation why there is limited work to address the social and structural influences of health could be that occupational therapists and related professionals in Zimbabwe are frustrated in a system that does not recognise them, and does not provide the conditions for them to achieve their goals with their clients - no provision for assistive devices, no support for work/home adaptations, no support for home/work visits (Dangarembizi et al, 2011), no sheltered workshops, inadequate vocational training centres, inadequate rehabilitation facilities for substance abusers and children, no vibrant CBR projects, among other issues. Occupational therapists have tried to address these issues in various ways which are highlighted later in the chapter.

In addition, there are other possible reasons why less attention and funding is given to social inclusion, such as, the state of the economy, the health market for private providers not being able to afford these services or the way in which national resources are distributed that does not prioritise social inclusion. Occupational therapists need to demonstrate the cost-effectiveness of their interventions. Furthermore, governments have to be persuaded that occupational therapy is important.

Some of the professional apathy can be understood especially in settings with high attrition rates among health personnel, and where departments are led by inadequately experienced graduates who are also planning to leave to other countries where there is better recognition and higher remuneration. From the issues highlighted above, it seems clear that there are multiple reasons why occupational therapists are predominantly working in acute settings. However, that results in some of the occupational needs of individuals, communities and populations not being addressed adequately, leading to high risk of social exclusion.

Recently, occupational therapists in Zimbabwe have been making efforts to promote social inclusion in different communities in addition to their traditional medically aligned services. For example, occupational therapists and occupational therapy students have been volunteering in new areas of practice and those areas that have not had an occupational therapist for some time, and these include schools and vocational rehabilitation centres. Also, the Zimbabwean Association of Occupational Therapists (ZAOT) managed to revive some occupational therapy services in rehabilitation institutions. These include clinical services and income generating projects. Community engagement, campaigns and partnerships with organisations such as Young Africa (an NGO which is geared towards youth empowerment and development) were also initiated in 2014 through the national association and the University of Zimbabwe rehabilitation department. These have been very instrumental in raising community awareness on human rights and legislation/policies that support vulnerable populations, as well as life skills training and youth empowerment. Of note, on the 2015 World Occupational Therapy Day, the national association partnered with the University of Zimbabwe, parliamentarians and DPOs to start an income generating project for people with learning disabilities at one of the rehabilitation centres.

Research on legislation and policy in promoting occupational therapy has intensified since 2013 when Zimbabwe hosted the Occupational Therapy African Regional Group (OTARG) congress. Some examples of research related to social inclusion undertaken by occupational therapists since September 2013 are: the USAID/CBM funded wheelchair user satisfaction and function (Visagie et al, 2015; 2016), study on the legislative and policy framework for occupational therapy practice in schools (Maphosa, 2014), outcome measures in line with national and international development blueprints like the Zimbabwe Agenda for Sustainable Socio-Economic Transformation (ZIMASSET) (Mataswa, 2016), and the extent to which UZ infrastructure is accessible to students with disabilities (Chigova, 2015).

We are proposing a framework that can be used to develop programmes that promote social inclusion in different communities. Outlined below is the framework and the proposed steps that occupational therapists and stakeholders can take to facilitate social inclusion (Table 2). This is work in progress based on our experiences during community based rural attachments for BSc Honours in Occupational Therapy and BSc Honours in Physiotherapy students at the University of Zimbabwe. This also borrows from Galvaan and Peters' Occupation-based Community Development Framework (2014). This will be an iterative process and will be tested on communities served by our students during their community based field attachments. Implementation of this framework will be spearheaded by the University training department through lectures and field attachment projects by students in collaboration with government ministries, DPOs and NGOs.

Table 2
Occupation-based Social Inclusion Framework

Step	Activities and outcomes
Identify a marginalised group or community at risk of social exclusion	Profile the occupational needs of the group or community Identify areas in which they experience exclusion from occupational participation in community Determine the extent of exclusion Identify the exclusionary factors
Scanning the legislative and policy environment	Do an audit of the international and national legislature supporting social inclusion Explore the level of implementation of the legislature and policy within this population Identify gaps in implementation of current legislation/policies Identify possible reasons for gaps in implementation When legislation is not available, advocate for establishment of such.
Identify key stakeholders in addressing the social inclusion	Possible key stakeholders - DPOs, community leaders, politicians, church organisations, NGOs and other professionals Form collaborations with these key stakeholders to address the presenting problems.
Design a programme (in collaboration with the community and key stakeholders) to promote social inclusion making use of the available legislation.	Open dialogue with key stakeholders Design programmes for raising awareness on current legislation and advocate for additional legislation that support social inclusion based on identified gaps In collaboration with key stakeholders design an occupation based programme that is acceptable in the community e.g. income generating projects and skills training Develop implementation strategies for the proposed programme Quantify the required resources and identify sources for them
Implementation of the occupation based social inclusion programme	The designed occupation based programme is implemented through participatory action approaches.
Monitoring and evaluation	Collect and keep comprehensive records/data Analyse the data Draw conclusions on the intervention aspects: Relevance, Effectiveness, Efficiency, Impact and Sustainability

Conclusion

Occupation-based social inclusion is a worthy means and end to addressing health and social challenges of marginalised groups including people with disabilities. However, for inclusion to be realised, there is need for relevant legislative and policy frameworks to be in place. Zimbabwe is well positioned in terms of the required legislative framework in the form of the national Constitution and several Acts of Parliament. Implementation of the available legislation can remain a pipe dream due to limited resources and a lack of implementation strategy; however, occupational therapists can take realistic steps towards implementation even with limited resources.

The process of tackling occupation-based social inclusion requires one to have a basic understanding of relevant legislation and an awareness of conventions that one's country is signatory to and legislation that is relevant. One step forward is curriculum review that takes up social inclusion as a human rights issue and emphasises legislation as part of context. Although the current University of Zimbabwe occupational therapy curriculum addressed the issue to some extent through courses like Applied Rehabilitation, we feel there is need for an explicit inclusion of the subject. Qualified therapists can be awarded continuing professional development points for attending short courses run through the national association on the subject. Recently, there has been an increased emphasis on social inclusion and the biopsychosocial model during training, i.e. clinical and community field attachments. Although examiners have been evaluating students on the aspect, we propose that a section on social inclusion and community reintegration be added to the case study guide for students and on the clinical practice evaluation form to ensure that every student/therapist addresses it for every client.

In recent years, occupational therapists have undertaken several steps to increase their understanding of national and international legislative and policy frameworks that support the inclusion and community reintegration of vulnerable populations like children and adults with disabilities. By embracing the national and international legislative and policy frameworks, occupational therapists in Zimbabwe are working on ways to increase their engagement with key stakeholders such as government ministries, Universities and DPOs in translating the UNCRPD into practice, training and research. This is critical in facilitating implementation or advocating for the country to ratify other relevant international legislations to which it may not yet be signatory. The issues raised above clearly point to the responsibility of occupational therapists in advancing their cause, and we have set out a framework and critical steps that occupational therapists can take to achieve the goal of occupation-based social inclusion. In all this, let the primary goal be service to the people, that is, improved access, empowerment, quality of life and inclusion.

References

Armstrong, D. (2002) The politics of self-advocacy and people with learning difficulties. *Policy & Politics*, 30, 3, 333-345

Chigova, (2015) *To what extent is the University of Zimbabwe infrastructure accessible to students with disabilities?* Unpublished BSc Hons dissertation submitted to the University of Zimbabwe.

Dangarembizi, N., Mlambo, T. and Chinhengo, T. (2011) Home visits by occupational therapists in Zimbabwe: The extent and challenges. *Central African Journal of Medicine*, 57, S18

Davys, D. and Tickle, E.J. (2008) Social inclusion and valued roles: A supportive framework. *International Journal of Therapy and Rehabilitation*, 15, 2–7

Fowler, F.C. (2000) *Policy studies for educational leaders: An introduction.* Upper Saddle River, NJ: Merrill Prentice Hall

Gannon, B. and Nolan, B. (2007) Impact of disability transitions on social inclusion. *Social Science and Medicine*, 64, 1425-1437

Galvaan, R. and Peters, L. (2014) *Occupation-based Community Development Framework.* University of Cape Town, Open Education Resource. [Accessed 7 September 2017 at https://vula.uct.ac.za/access/content/group/9c29ba04-b1ee-49b9-8c85-9a468b556ce2/OBCDF/index.html]

Kenyon, S. (2003) Understanding social exclusion and social inclusion. *Proceedings of the ICE-Municipal Engineer*, 156, 2, 97-104

Joubert, R.W. (2010) *Indigenous fruits from exotic roots?: Revisiting the South African occupational therapy curriculum* (Doctoral dissertation). South Africa: University of Kwazulu- Natal [Accessed 7 September 2017 at https://researchspace.ukzn.ac.za/handle/10413/862]

Knight, J. (2004) Internationalization remodelled: Definition, approaches, and rationales. *Journal of Studies in International Education*, 8, 1, 5–31

Kuo, A. (2011) A transactional view: Occupation as a means to create experiences that matter. *Journal of Occupational Science* 18, 131–138

Kupe, W. and Mazula, S. (2010) *Federation of Organisations of Disabled people in Zimbabwe (FODPZ) Country Report.* [Accessed 7 September 2017 https://assets.publishing.service.gov.uk/media/57a08afee5274a31e00008d6/Zimbabwe.v1.pdf]

Leclair, L.L.(2010) Re-examining concepts of occupation and occupation-based models: Occupational therapy and community development. *Canadian. Journal of Occupational. Therapy* 77, 15-21

Levers, L., Magweva, F.I. and Mufema, E. (2010) *Poverty Levels Among People With Disabilities: An evaluation of the need for developing a disability social protection scheme in Zimbabwe. Final Report.* Harare, Zimbabwe: NASCOH

Magweva, F., Mpofu, E., Ngazimbi, E., Anwer,J., Brooks, J., & Johnson, E. (2012) Issues of vulnerability. in L. L. Levers (Ed) *Trauma Counseling: Theories and interventions.* New York: Springer Publishing Company. New York.

Maphosa, (2014) *Legislative framework for the provision of occupational therapy services in public schools in Zimbabwe.* Unpublished BSc Hons dissertation submitted to the University of Zimbabwe

Mataswa, (2016) *Outcome measures and the factors associated with targeted outcomes in Occupational Therapy Mental Health practice in Zimbabwe.* Unpublished BSc Hons dissertation submitted to the University of Zimbabwe

Mlambo, T., Munambah, N., Nhunzvi, C. and Murambidzi, I. (2014) Mental Health Services in Zimbabwe - a case of Zimbabwe National Association of Mental Health. *World Federation of Occupational Therapists Bulletin*, 70, 1, 18-21.

Munemo, E. and Tom, T. (2013) Effectiveness of existing legislation in empowering people with disabilities. *Global Advanced Research Journal of Educational Research and Review*, 2, 2, 31-40

Pal, J., Vartak, A., Vyas, V., Chatterjee, S., Paisios, N. and Cherian, R. (2010) *A ratification of means: International law and assistive technology in the developing world.* in: Proceedings of the 4th ACM/IEEE International Conference on Information and Communication Technologies and Development. [Accessed 7 September 2017 at https://pdfs.semanticscholar. org/f41a/a788f2e81ecfbe7f2ec3b644a27f57f87a85.pdf]

Parliament of Zimbabwe (1972) *Children's Act: Chapter 5: 06.* [Accessed 7 September 2017 at http://www.parlzim.gov.zw/acts-list/childrens-act-5-06]

Parliament of Zimbabwe (1985) *Labour Act: Chapter 28: 01.* [Accessed 7 September 2017 at http://www.ilo.org/dyn/natlex/docs/ELECTRONIC/1850/76997/F2029058807/ ZWE1850%202005.pdf]

Parliament of Zimbabwe (1987) *Education Act: Chapter 25:04.* [Accessed 7 September 2017 at http://www.parlzim.gov.zw/acts-list/education-act-25-04]

Parliament of Zimbabwe (1992a) *Disabled Persons Act: Chapter 17: 01.* [Accessed 7 September 2017 at http://www.parlzim.gov.zw/acts-list/disabled-persons-act-17-01]

Parliament of Zimbabwe (1992b) *Land Acquisition Act: Chapter 20: 10.* [Accessed 7 September 2017 at http://www.parlzim.gov.zw/acts-list/land-acquisition-act-20-10]

Parliament of Zimbabwe (1995) *War Veterans Act: Chapter 11: 15.* [Accessed 7 September 2017 at http://www.ilo.org/dyn/natlex/docs/ELECTRONIC/101333/122039/F14595782/ ZWE101333.pdf]

Parliament of Zimbabwe (1996) *Mental Health Act: Chapter 15:12.* [Accessed 7 September 2017 at http://www.parlzim.gov.zw/acts-list/mental-health-act-15-12]

Parliament of Zimbabwe (2008) *Indigenization and Economic Empowerment Act: Chapter 14: 33.* [Accessed 7 September 2017 at http://www.eisourcebook.org/cms/January%20 2016/Zimbabwe%20Indigenisation%20and%20Economic%20Empowerment%20Act.pdf]

Parliament of Zimbabwe (2013) *Constitution of Zimbabwe Amendment (No. 20) Act, 2013.* [Accessed 7 September 2017 at http://www.wipo.int/edocs/lexdocs/laws/en/zw/zw038en. pdf]

Russell, A. and Lloyd, C. (2004) Partnerships in mental health: Addressing barriers to social inclusion. *International Journal of Therapy and Rehabilitation.* 11, 267–74

Samyshkin, Y., Huxley, P. and Atun, R. (2010) Rehabilitation and social inclusion of people with mental illness in Russia. *Psychiatric Services*, 61,3, 222-224

Schneider, M., Eide, A.H., Amin, M., MacLachlan, M. and Mannan, H. (2013) Inclusion of vulnerable groups in health policies: Regional policies on health priorities in Africa, *African Journal of Disability* 2, 1

Smith, T.B. (1973) The policy implementation process. *Policy Sciences.* 4, 2, 197–209

Townsend, E. and Wilcock, A.A. (2004) Occupational justice and client-centred practice: A dialogue in progress. *Canadian Journal of Occupational Therapy* 71, 75–87

United Nations (1989) *The United Nations Convention on the rights of the child.* [Accessed 30 November 2016 at http://www.ohchr.org/en/professionalinterest/pages/crc.aspx]

United Nations (2006) *Convention on the Rights of Persons with Disabilities* [Accessed 17 January 2011 at http://www.un.org/disabilities/convention/conventionfull.shtml]

United Nations (2015) Definition of key terms used in the UN Treaty Collection [online]. [Accessed 28 May 2015 at https://treaties.un.org/Pages/overview.aspx?path=overview/definition/page1_en.xml]

Visagie, S., Mlambo, T., van der Veen, J., Nhunzvi, C., Tigere, D. and Scheffler, E. (2015) Is any wheelchair better than no wheelchair? A Zimbabwean perspective. *African Journal of Disability*, 4, 1, 1-10

Visagie, S., Mlambo, T., van der Veen, J., Nhunzv, C., Tigere, D. and Scheffler, E. (2016) Impact of structured wheelchair services on satisfaction and function of wheelchair users in Zimbabwe. *African Journal of Disability*, 5, 1, 1-11

Whiteford, G. and Pereira, R. (2012) Occupation, inclusion and participation. in G. Whiteford and C. Hocking (Eds.) *Occupational Science: Social inclusion, participation.* London: Wiley-Blackwell (pp.188-207)

WHO, ILO, and IDDC UNESCO. (2010) *Community-based rehabilitation: CBR Guidelines.* Geneva, Switzerland

Wilcock, A. A. (2006) *An occupational perspective of health.* Thorofare, NJ: Slack

Chapter 6
Rights based approaches to inclusion and rehabilitation: From individual stories to collective actions

Rocco Angarola and Krishna Gautam

Introduction to CIL – Kathmandu

CIL-Kathmandu (Independent Living Centre - CIL) is a completely non-profitable and non-political (i.e. not aligned to any political party) self-help organisation entirely run by persons with disabilities. It is a non-governmental organisation established to work for the promotion and protection of the rights of persons with disabilities (PWDs) through the concept of independent living. The term *Independent Living* as defined by people with disabilities does not mean doing things for yourself, or living on your own. It means having choice and control over the assistance and/ or equipment/assistive devices needed for daily life and having access to amenities that society has to offer such as housing, transport, health services, employment, as well as entertainment, education and training opportunities. Independent living is a vision, a philosophy and a movement of persons with disabilities to promote and protect the human rights of PWDs. It interprets disability in the social model and a rights-based approach. The concept of independent living was born in Berkeley University, California, USA in the 1970s (Willig Levy, 1998), the movement spread to Europe and Asia in the 1980s, and has since reached around the globe and changed the way people view and respond to disability.

In Nepal, CIL-Kathmandu has been working in policy advocacy for increasing the participation of PWDs in the decision making process, peer counseling with disabled persons, personal assistant services (PAS), and independent living programmes (ILP) in terms of training in daily living skills etc.

History of the foundation of CIL-Kathmandu

As an organisation CIL-Kathmandu started its work on disability rights in 2005. The first initiative to promote the concept of independent living in Nepal was brought to disabled persons with the leadership of Mr. Krishna Gautam (a person with physical disabilities). When Mr. Gautam came back to Nepal after the completion of a ten month Duskin Leadership Training, a programme for people with disabilities in Japan (Duskin n.d.), he undertook this initiative with the support of some other experienced and energetic disabled youth. Since Mr. Gautam had gained a good knowledge of the independent living concept during his period of training he was enthusiastic to promote it in Nepal. The main objective behind this effort was to shift the paradigm of disability from charity-based, and thus based in dependency, to rights-based independence.

Photo 1: Barrier Free Campaign run annually by CIL Kathmandu

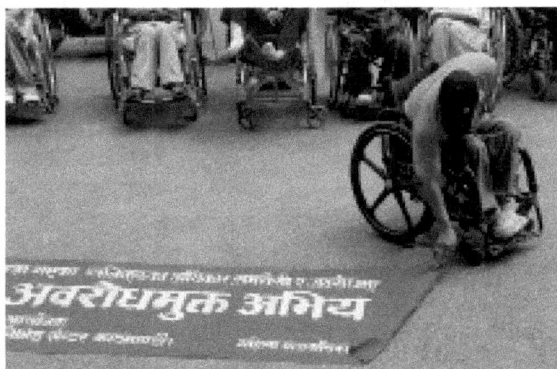

In 2005 the Nepali political situation was not favourable for the work of a rights-based movement. The whole nation was suffering from a phase of extreme armed conflict and was under direct rule by the King. Through the leadership of a seven party alliance (which aimed to develop a federal democratic state) the people of Nepal prepared a peoples' movement to liberate the country from autocracy. In this situation CIL-Kathmandu also wanted to show its solidarity with the movement through the physical involvement of persons with disabilities. In April 2006 all Nepalese came onto the streets to agitate against the situation and CIL-Kathmandu also showed its bold contribution to the movement on behalf of civil society by involving PWDs in the great peoples' movement.

After the success of the peoples' movement CIL-Kathmandu was legally registered in the district administration office Kathmandu, in August 2006, along with the changing political scenario.

Collaborations, partnerships and alliances

Relationship with civil society

CIL-Kathmandu, as an organisation, has always believed in collaboration. Therefore, it has maintained relationships and joined together with other organisations, alliances and forums to achieve various common objectives about a range of social issues. For example it is a member of the Federation of Democratic NGOs, of the Human Rights Joint Forum and of the Citizen Movement for Democracy and Peace Nepal.

Relationship with the Government

As a result of the organisation's active involvement in the democracy movement in 2006, the Nepali Government recognised CIL-Kathmandu as one of the key stakeholders to work jointly on disability rights. It also has a regular partnership with the Ministry of Women, Children and Social Welfare and the Social Welfare Council. It has been providing feedback and suggestions on disability issues to the pioneer government agencies such as the National Planning Commission, Ministry of Finance, Ministry of Peace and Reconstruction, Kathmandu Metropolitan City, District Development Committee Kathmandu, and the District Development Committee Lalipur.

Relationship with the International Community

CIL-Kathmandu has also links with a large number of international organisations. For example CIL-Kathmandu is a Member of the Asia Pacific Network of Independent Living (APNIL), and is associated with the Duskin Ainowa Foundation Japan and with Blue Law International and Human Rights - Yes! in America. In addition CIL-Kathmandu has short term or event based partnerships with a range of organisations, for example, Save the Children Norway and USA.

Vision, mission and goals of the organisation

In accordance with the concept of independent living, the organisation believes in the value of community-based, stake-holder controlled services, support, resources and skill training. This work, importantly developed and controlled by the people themselves, enables people with disabilities to live 'normal' lives in the community. The organisation recognises and its work is characterised by the principles of Independent Living. Based on human rights it is recognised that there should be no segregation due to disability or stereotype, no institutionalisation, and it should be recognised that PWDs are not sick and do not necessarily need help from medical professions for daily living. The importance of self-help is recognised, that people learn and grow from discussing their needs, concerns and issues with people with similar experiences, that they are able to decide which service may be most useful for them, and that the most useful services are those that are managed and operated by persons with disability. In order for these to be achieved systemic, long-term and community-wide activities, advocating for change are required, while full participation in the community requires the removal of multiple barriers including the physical and social. Finally the organisation supports cross-disability approaches where people with different types of disability work for the benefit of all. The organisation has developed its vision, mission and goals in line with these values (see Table 1).

Table 1. Vision, Mission and Goals of CIL-Kathmandu

Vision: Empowered and productive persons with disabilities living with dignity and independently with the full realization of human rights in a barrier free environment and chosen community.

Mission: Promotion and strengthening values, principles and practices of Independent Living throughout the Nation.

Goal: CIL-Kathmandu has set the following goals to reach its mission:
- Establish and strengthen IL centers as the key mediators of government to implement IL programs.
- Obtain state and social responsibility for the promotion and development of IL Programs.
- Achieve adoption of anti-discriminatory laws, policies regarding the rights of PWDs and their effective implementation.

Objective and activities

CIL-Kathmandu is committed to enabling the participation of PWD's at the social, political, economic, physical, and cultural level to maintain their livelihood with their self-esteem, independence and dignity. The main goal is for all PWDs to have the opportunity to participate and to be active members of their communities. There are four main barriers that PWDs face everywhere and that the organisation wants to overcome. These are: attitudinal barriers; architectural barriers; communication barriers; and institutional barriers.

CIL-Kathmandu encourages PWD to come out on the streets to make their voices heard in order to change the attitudes of non-disabled people and to advocate for the development of policies and programmes from the Government (see Photos 1 and 2). CIL-Kathmandu has developed regular engagement and negotiation with civic society, professional bodies, national and international stakeholders as well as local and central government.

Photo 2: Disability Rights campaigning activities organised by CIL every year in Kathmandu

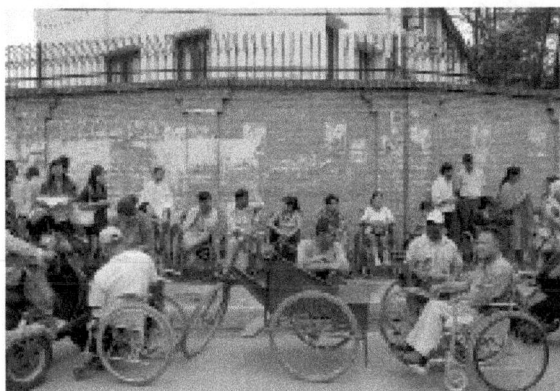

The organisation's core activities are: advocacy programmes; peer support counselling; independent living programmes aimed at gaining specific daily living skills and vocational skills required to live independently; support in the transition to independent living; assistive technology services; and ongoing campaigning for the promotion and protection of the rights of people with disabilities.

The activities of CIL-Kathmandu are supported financially by a range of organisations, these include the government of Nepal, various ministries and municipalities, the Kathmandu university and other institutions, together with various organisations in Japan. There is an executive committee, an advisory committee, a number of salaried staff and a large number of volunteers.

Activities of CIL-Kathmandu

CIL-Kathmandu has organised a wide range of activities, many run as programmes in collaboration with a range of national and international organisations. Some examples of these are (CIL-Kathmandu, 2011):

Monthly independent living discussion programme

This was developed in collaboration with Action Aid Nepal. Key activities of this programme are monthly activities to raise awareness of disability and independent living with a range of stakeholders, such as professionals, NGOs, Government authorities, the media, parents.

Promotion and development of the independent living concept in Nepal

This programme is developed in collaboration with the Mainstream Association Japan since 2006. Key activities include work to expand the network of CIL and the personal assistant service, together with administrative support.

Promotion and protection of rights of PWDs through advocacy and independent living activities

This programme ran in collaboration with the Ministry of Women, Children and Social Welfare, from 2007 to 2009. Activities included advocacy and lobbying; peer counseling to build self-confidence; providing practical knowledge and training to disabled people on daily living skills.

CIL-Kathmandu has also established the *Manufacture of the Standard Manual Wheelchairs* for PWDs in Nepal with the support of donors from the UK. It has also established an *Education Fund* to support children disabilities in various districts of Nepal.

Some important outputs observed as the result of CIL's work

There are some significant achievements which have really supported the promotion of disability rights in Nepal. The regular, joint and hard effort of disabled people and their self-help organisations are the key reasons behind these achievements. CIL-Kathmandu has always taken a decisive and important role in leading this joint movement since its establishment. Since 2013 we have observed some significant achievements in policy and practices of government for promoting the rights of disabled people. These include:

The contribution of PWDs in the great Peoples' Movement of 2006 has been highly valued by political parties, civil society and the international communities as well. CIL-Kathmandu has played a leading role in making PWDs visible in the peoples' movement from the side of civil society. The Nepal government has signed the United Nations Convention on the Rights of Persons with Disabilities (UNCRPD) in 2010.

Because of the regular campaign carried out by CIL-Kathmandu and other organisations for a barrier free environment, including actively refusing to accept the non-accessible public building, some of the government buildings such as the Ministry of Finance, Ministry of Home, Ministry of Physical Planning and Construction, Ministry of Information and Communication, Ministry of Tourism, National Planning Commission, and the House of Representatives have been accommodated with wheelchair ramps. Similarly, some District Administration Offices, District Development Offices in some districts, banks, some other public buildings, parks and other newly constructed building have also made wheel chair ramps in the main entrance of the building (Photo 3).

Photo 3: A ramp facilitating wheel chair access

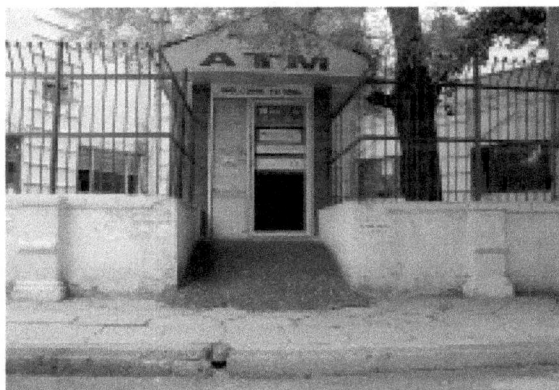

A number of financial benefits have been achieved for PWDs. The Central Government of Nepal has allocated Disability Allowances of Rs.1000 per month for persons having severe disabilities and has increased the rate for other categories to Rs.300 per month. The Government of Nepal has also announced a 100% tax exemption for those specially adapted scooters (converted from petrol driven models) which are used by disabled people for their private mobility. There is a 45% discount in public transport fares and a 50% discount in domestic air fares for PWDs. In addition the Local Government of Nepal (district development committee) has introduced a provision for 1 - 5% of the total district's budget to be allocated for the development of disabled people, under the Local Self Governance Act (HM Government, Nepal, 1999).

Of considerable significance is that the Central Government of Nepal allocated Rs. 10.000.000 to work for the promotion of the rights and for the betterment of disabled people in the budget of fiscal year 2015/2016. This amount is the largest fund ever allocated for disabled people in the country's history. The National Budget of Nepal has addressed the activities of CIL-Kathmandu and allocated some funds which will be used in following areas: advocacy; peer counseling; attendant services; independent living programmes; and barrier free campaigning.

Further achievements include that the Interim Constitution of Nepal 2006 has addressed the need for the inclusion of PWDs in the state mechanisms and policy making level as well. Because of the regular interventions of CIL-Kathmandu the Constitution Assembly (CA) directory has ensured the provisions of a sign language interpreter for deaf CA members and a personal assistant for wheelchair user CA member representatives to CA. It is also important to note here that two persons from the disabled community Mr. Raghabir Joshi (with a hearing impairment) and Ms. Indira Gurung (with a physical disability) have been nominated as CA members. Similarly the directory has also ensured the provisions for two disabled people to participate in the main committee to be formed for the drafting of the constitution.

At an organisational level CIL-Kathmandu has established 9 IL Centers in different parts of Nepal. They are launching a variety of IL activities.

Contemporary issues

The 2015 earthquake in Nepal has done significant damage to the country and its infrastructure, and has had a huge influence on subsequent events. The impact, which will be felt over a considerable time in the future, was illustrated by the presentation given by Krishna Gautam; Secretary General CIL-Kathmandu, at the VDAH day in December 2015:

> Nepal was devastated by a massive earthquake on the 25th April 2015. Many areas were severely affected (destroyed), including the Kathmandu Valley, Shindupalzu, Gurka Nagarkot amongst others.
>
> Consequently many people have been affected. More than 8,856 people were killed, and 22,309 were injured (Associated Press, 2016). Early reports following the earthquake indicated that approximately 1 in 3 of those injured would require follow-up rehabilitation treatment (WHO, 2015). According to the latest status released by the National Federation of the Disabled Nepal there have been around 400 people who have suffered spinal cord injury (Livability, 2016).

Right after the earthquake many people were admitted to hospitals in order to get treatment. Upon discharge they did not have anywhere to go in the community to receive rehabilitation for their spinal cord injury. There are some Rehabilitation Centres in Kathmandu, where people initially received treatments such as physiotherapy. However, after three months they were required to go back to their homes and to their communities. They then faced a variety of problems, for example, suffering from diseases and bed sores, they did not have appropriate wheelchairs, and they did not have any types of assistive devices. This resulted in a variety of challenges for those who live in their communities. To tackle these challenges CIL-Kathmandu has created a Rescue and Relief programme.

In June 2015 CIL established an earthquake relief camp for PWDs at Jawalakhel sports ground. At the camp there were around 80 PWDs including children. The camp provided shelter, food, clean water, medications, and some assistive devices. However, in the beginning of this programme CIL-Kathmandu and the disabled community faced many challenges due to the inaccessibility of the physical environment, including no accessible toilets. After that, with the support of Red Cross Society, this camp was relocated to the Chassle area, where the environment was made accessible and CIL built accessible tents and toilets to accommodate PWDs. This camp was organised and managed by CIL for four months. After that, CIL provided wheelchairs and other assistive devices to PWDs. Upon the closure of the camp, CIL supported people to get back to their homes and communities.

Many International Non-Governmental Organisations (INGOs) and the Government of Nepal were planning to build an institution to accommodate those who had become severely injured after the earthquake. CIL opposed this plan because we believe that there are no human rights in institutions. For this reason, we asked the international community to support our peers to go back to their homes, families and communities. The campaign had success, and for this reason people who stayed at the relief camp returned to live in their communities. At present CIL is providing them with personal assistant (support workers) services, appropriate assistive devices, for example wheelchairs, an allowance to cover the costs of accommodation, and we are also providing support to seek employment. As a result they are able to live more meaningful lives in the community.

The earthquake resulted in an increased number of people with disabilities. We are still facing many difficulties in a variety of areas. We believe that these can be best resolved by a joint effort from the local and international communities. Locally CIL- Kathmandu with the support of National Federation of the Disabled Nepal, UNDP and some Governmental offices, have organised a donor meeting. The purpose of this meeting is to request our donors to develop specific programmes in the disability field. For example, as well as a rescue centre and a shelter camp, the creation of Rehabilitation Centres where PWDs can receive treatments from a full range of medical disciplines and Allied Health Professions. Furthermore we believe that the variety of allied health professions will play a key role in delivering, in partnership with persons with disability, creative solutions that will support maximum independence and quality of life. In addition we need to ensure the provision of assistive devices e.g. appropriate wheelchairs, as pivotal to our independence and fundamental to our rights as citizens.

At the same time our ongoing work to ensure the full participation of all requires us to continue our work, and we are appealing to the international community and the Nepal Government to make the man-made infrastructure accessible, disabled friendly. This will allow all PWDs to increase their mobility and participation. We are also requesting our Government to develop employment services for PWDs. In the absence of this the Government has to support social security since many people with profound and severe disabilities are still confined within their homes. This occurs because of lack of support such as assistive devices, limited accessibility etc.

We can conclude that although in 2010 the Government of Nepal ratified the UNCRPD, at the time of writing policies were still not implemented. We believe that we have to develop national domestic laws and legislations to support PWDs and the victims of the earthquake. We are requesting the international community to develop a programme and policies to support PWDs. We believe that we are the most vulnerable group, most backward community, where a lot of work is needed. We believe that allied health professions can provide a fundamental role in supporting PWDS. Hence their support will be very important to improve the quality of life of PWDS, to live with dignity and to enable each individual to flourish in their own community. We would like to participate in every aspect of life and have the power to make our own decisions.

Photo 4: CIL members visiting accessible public places in Pokara

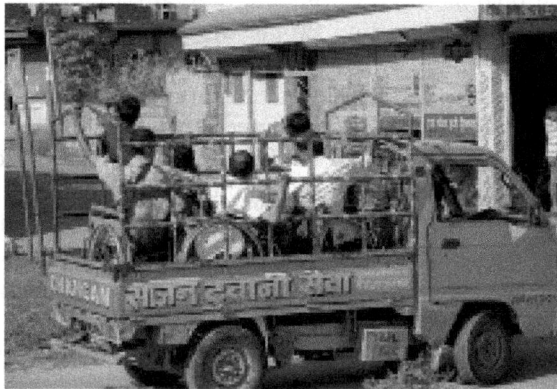

Conclusion

The earthquake of 2015 increased the number of people living with disability in Nepal, which has stretched the already limited resources. At the same time the need for people with disability to maintain their right to self-advocacy and to live independently needs to be constantly upheld. CIL-Kathmandu, with its active membership, continues to take part in wide-spread campaigns to promote accessibility for PWD (see for example http://cil.org.np/en/). However, the importance of partnership working between CIL-Kathmandu and national and international organisations and funders is evident throughout the development of the CIL-Kathmandu since it was founded in 2005, but particularly for the work that is needed to support the recently increased number of people with disability. Developing such partnerships to support and implement a variety of projects will remain a priority for the organisation in the coming years.

References

Associated Press (2016) A list of some effects from Nepal's earthquake 1 year ago. *Mail on line*. 21 April [Accessed 13 October 2016 at http://www.dailymail.co.uk/wires/ap/article-3551129/A-list-effects-Nepals-earthquake-1-year-ago.html]

Duskin Leadership Training in Japan (n.d.) [Accessed 7 May 2016 at http://www.normanet.ne.jp/~duskin/english/index.html]

HM Government, Nepal (1999) *Local Self-Governance ACT, 2055*. Nepal: Ministry of Law and Justice Law Books Management Board [Accessed 7 September 2017 at http://www.np.undp.org/content/dam/nepal/docs/reports/governance/UNDP_NP_Local%20Self-Governance%20Act%201999,%20MoLJ,HMG.pdf]

Livability (2016) *The Nepal Earthquakes: One year on*. [Accessed 13 October 2016 at http://www.livability.org.uk/nepal-earthquake-one-year-on/] National Federation of the Disabled (2016) *Earthquake 2015*. [Accessed 30 November 2016 at http://www.nfdn.org.np/search

Willig C.L. (1998) *A people's history of the Independent Living Movement*. Independent Living Institute. [Accessed 15 September 2016 at www.independentliving.org/docs5/ILhistory.html]

World Health Organisation (2015) *WHO mobilises funds for long-term spinal cord treatment after Nepal earthquake: News release 2 May* [Accessed at http://www.who.int/mediacentre/news/releases/2015/mobilizing-funds-nepal/en/]

Section 7
Participatory approaches and research

This section introduces innovative ways of knowing and engaging with people to take part in research, and the idea of research as occupation. The first three chapters particularly focus on ways of knowing, co-creation and creative approaches to understanding. Their innovative approaches to presenting their discussion is in itself a stimulus for broadening perspectives while the richness of the polyphony of the authors perspectives is evident in the narratives. The final four chapters focus more on the research process itself, offering critical discussions of how research as occupation can be a site of exclusion, of inclusive research designs and processes, and illustrating research as opportunities for advocacy and change. Again the multiple perspectives offered by the writing (and research) teams provide rich opportunities for reflection and future action.

In the first chapter Crawford, McCallum and an anonymous author, writing from Australia, present the process of story-telling as a tool for developing connections, understandings and so enable more inclusive communities. They present both theoretical perspectives and an example of developing and telling a story about the experience of being an asylum-seeker.

Chamberlain and Craig present a very different approach in employing design to engage people in research and to have a voice regarding their needs and choices for meaningful occupation. Particularly focusing on older people who can be disenfranchised and stigmatised by society, through case studies they demonstrate their involvement in the studies of Lab4Living, UK and the process of overcoming barriers due to language, culture, gender and age.

Burger's chapter takes us to the world of the clinic and the struggle for service user voices and representation in the decision making structures of mental health services. She describes the research of the client council in one large organisation and the resulting innovative feed-back system that was developed and eventually implemented by the Dutch government to ensure engagement.

Focusing in more detail on the research process Laliberte Rudman and co-authors share the results of a Canadian photovoice project with First Nation youth. These young people are engaged in an exploration of their journeys in post-secondary education using a culturally respectful approach. This chapter invites consideration not only of the research process itself but also the purpose of the research in leading to change and development in institutional structures and processes.

Layton, Buchanan and Wilson continue the focus on the research process, suggesting the value of considering research itself as an occupation, and thereby who may be included and excluded from such occupation. They challenge some of the traditional approaches to research and provide rich insights into what enabling research as an inclusive occupation might look like.

Finally, Piškur et al, continue this discussion of citizen participation in research, providing rich illustrations from a research project involving parents as co-researchers, and suggesting ways in which higher educational institutions may support researchers to be more participative in their approaches.

Chapter 7
Storytelling:
A tool for occupational therapists, especially when working with asylum seekers

Emma Crawford, Alexandra McCallum, and Anonymous

Living creatively with problems can be an alternative to 'fixing' people and situations (Westoby & Dowling, 2009). Perhaps this is an apt tactic when working with asylum seekers, whose situations are difficult to 'fix'. They have unfulfilled human rights (Campbell & Steel, 2015), are socially excluded in their home countries and their host countries (Hynes, 2011), and are situated within complex global migration structures (Stewart, 2008). Storytelling is a creative tool that occupational therapists might use with people whose barriers to occupational engagement expand beyond individual concerns to include harming social structures with no immediate fix. Storytelling creates connections and through the telling and re-telling of stories more socially inclusive communities can be created.

Asylum seekers, occupational deprivation and social inclusion

Asylum seekers are different to other migrants. They are allowed to apply for a refugee protection visa on arrival in their host country because they will be persecuted if they remain in their home countries while they wait for their refugee applications to be processed (Raveendran, 2012; Price, 2010; Field, 2006). While they wait for their visas to be processed, asylum seekers are segregated from the communities in their host countries because they are non-citizens who arrived without visas (Campbell & Steel, 2015; Hynes, 2011). Other migrants, including refugees, are required to organise their visas before leaving their homes to live elsewhere for safety, work, family, health, economic, or other reasons and are thus subject to more inclusive conditions.

Asylum seekers can be seen as occupationally deprived (Morville et al, 2014; Morville & Erlandsson, 2013; Burchett & Matheson, 2010, Steindl et al, 2008; Connor Schisler & Polatajko, 2002). This means that the systemic prejudice in the political, societal, and institutional environments surrounding asylum seekers precludes them from engaging in what is meaningful in their lives.

Asylum seekers are often excluded in the countries where they seek protection. This occurs through government measures to enforce of border protection and immigration control. As non-citizens in their host countries, asylum seekers are often segregated, isolated, and disadvantaged. They might be held in detention centres, sent outside the host country's borders where that country claims little responsibility for what happens to them, or placed in the community with little support and often prohibition from work (Kalt et al, 2013; Rosenberger & Konig, 2012; Andersson & Nilsson, 2011; Hynes, 2011; Kissoon, 2010). Such measures are intended to curb migration flows by excluding people fleeing harmful, life-threatening situations from community participation. Asylum seekers are socially excluded through the implementation of these policies. As a result they have little to do and are often precluded from engaging in what is meaningful to them (Campbell & Steel, 2015).

For asylum seekers, like many other disadvantaged groups, 'occupational deprivation is a by-product of social exclusion, and can therefore be addressed through policies and strategies that enable inclusion' (Whiteford, 2011, p.545). Given that social inclusion might be a possible antidote to occupational deprivation, this chapter presents storytelling as a mechanism for social inclusion for asylum seekers.

Storytelling and social inclusion

Stories of everyday life can be defined as repeatable sets of words (or actions or pictures) which explain personal experiences within a particular cultural context (Sakiyama et al, 2010; Clouston, 2003). There are many definitions and types of storytelling. This chapter takes the perspective that storytelling occurs naturally within everyday life, such as 'in a bar, a parking lot, or a supermarket aisle' (Tyler & Swarts, 2012, p.455). This type of storytelling involves a relational practice of sharing personal experiences in an emergent and sometimes non-linear conversational process which involves both listening and telling (Tyler & Swarts, 2012). Considering this definition, storytelling is occupational in nature; it is an activity that holds meaning and is carried out in a person's unique life context. Storytelling can contribute to social inclusion in two ways, through connection and through re-telling.

Initially, storytelling provides a shared communicative space between storyteller and listener (Westoby & Dowling, 2009). Within this space the teller and listener(s) begin to create connections, the foundation of community. To be connected is to be socially included.

For example, the organisation Scattered People in Australia engages in songwriting with asylum seekers to create opportunities for them to share their stories (Sweet Freedom Ltd, 2015). Cultural practices and norms are brought to Scattered People by asylum seekers, and these often form the basis of the songs. For example, in Persian culture, poetry and metaphors are common means of storytelling and self-expression so many Persian asylum seekers offer their poetry which becomes song lyrics. Connections are created at the gatherings where stories are shared, transformed into songs, and passed on over the years. This builds a supportive and inclusive community for the asylum seekers involved, volunteers who attend the gatherings, and community development practitioners who coordinate the gatherings. The importance of the connections and social inclusion created through this storytelling and songwriting group is illustrated in their song 'Need One Another', released in

2011 (Sweet Freedom Ltd, 2015) which describes asylum seekers needing others when feeling downhearted or low, to help move on from negative feelings or experiences. The song uses the metaphor of spring and the breakthrough of new life in relation to reaching out to others.

Secondarily, the re-telling of stories can influence broader social structures to create social change. As the echoes of stories resonate beyond their initial telling, societal attitudes might slowly shift and policies might begin to create socially inclusive conditions. Re-telling might occur directly from the storyteller to people she/he encounters, indirectly through the recounting of stories by the original listener, or widely through publishing. Storytelling can provide marginalised people with opportunities to articulate their experiences and may be a means for political engagement (Pollard, 2012). Additionally, publication can provide recognition and validation of experiences for marginalised people (Pollard, 2012). For example, stories might be shared as part of an advocacy strategy.

In the example of Scattered People, the group aims to combat negative media and political rhetoric by promoting attitudes of 'compassion and desire for fair treatment of fellow human beings' (Sweet Freedom Ltd, 2015). This is done through publishing albums. The organisation has developed and published three complete albums that provide a conduit for sharing individual stories with others who might be unconnected to those asylum seekers in any other way. Similarly, the Refugee Claimants Support Service (2006) in Queensland, Australia has also compiled an anthology of asylum seekers' stories, poems, experiences and recipes. This book, Alone Together, was used to promote awareness in society regarding asylum seekers' experiences as well as a tool for advocacy that was referred to by the organisation when promoting policy change to address unnecessary hardships imposed on asylum seekers by the government.

Storytelling in occupational therapy

Occupational therapists are called to 'work with groups, communities and societies to enhance participation in occupation for all persons' by the World Federation of Occupational Therapists (2011). Storytelling can be a starting point for fulfilling this mandate, imagining and generating opportunities for occupational engagement for people whose human rights have been breached, including asylum seekers. Clouston (2003) explains that storytelling can be a therapeutic modality to overcome barriers to occupational engagement, and create possibilities for change.

Occupational therapists see their clients' stories as sources of information for building relationships and informing practice (Bonsall, 2012; Sakiyama et al, 2010; Clouston, 2003; Mattingly & Lawlor, 2000; Price-Lackey & Cashman, 1996). Galheigo et al. (2012) promote listening to and using life-stories as a useful tool for occupational therapists to understand the perceptions of people with disabilities, which might influence their participation in family and community life.

Listening to stories of everyday life, for example asking a client about one day in their life or for their overarching life-story, creates a connection that helps occupational therapists understand meanings underpinning actions (Bonsall, 2012; Wright St

Clair, 2003). It elucidates historical, cultural and societal context (Mattingly, 1998). While caution should be taken not to over-interpret messages from stories, valuable lessons can be learned from them. Occupational therapists can understand people's experiences, meanings, and hopes through stories (Clouston, 2003; Mattingly, 1998; Polkinghorne, 1991).

Occupational therapists' engagement in storytelling can contribute to the way clients tell their stories, shaping the meanings made (Clouston, 2003). Guidance for storytellers to consider their experiences in new ways can change people's judgments themselves and their experiences. Through telling their own stories, people become aware of and able to transform their own realities (Galheigo et al, 2012). This was noted during the co-creation of the story presented below. Gentle facilitation for commencing, continuing, and delving deeper into stories can (as illustrated in this project) support shared understandings and opportunities for self-expression, when this might be difficult in other contexts (e.g. providing a medical history, or background information for a therapy session).

Storytelling allows for self-expression, new understandings, and ideas about possibilities for change. Often, occupational therapists ask clients for simple stories about their daily activities and routines. Wright St Clair (2003) described the creative use of storytelling with women with multiple sclerosis (MS), identifying metaphors describing MS as an aggressor, saviour, guest, partner, and adversary. She suggested that the occupation of storytelling allowed women with MS to express themselves, redefine meanings of life events, and engage in transformational processes that changed how they lived. Another example of storytelling in occupational therapy is the creation of fictional scenes and stories in sand-trays, peer validation of stories and experiences, and storybook making with children who have experienced trauma allowing opportunities for emotional expression, understanding, and acceptance (Scaletti & Hocking, 2010).

These examples demonstrate the many forms that stories can take. Personal stories of everyday life might contribute to concrete understandings of a person's life, and fictional stories might provide insights into emotional experiences, creating spaces for understanding and acceptance. Achieving understanding and acceptance can form the basis of genuine human connection and a starting point for social inclusion. Extension of the content of stories beyond the immediate therapy environment, for example sharing stories with wider communities or using stories as part of advocacy strategies, can create further connections and promote structural change for social inclusion (Westoby & Dowling, 2009).

The personal nature of storytelling and cautions for occupational therapists

Stories are personal (Scaletti & Hocking, 2010). Intimate details are abundant in stories, so storytelling, along with authentic listening, requires and builds trust, connection and thus inclusion. Appropriate therapist disclosure of their own personal stories can also provide information which clients may use to decide how much, or how little, they will place their trust in that therapist. Clouston (2003) warns therapists to be aware of ethical boundaries and personal care when engaging in storytelling practices. With asylum seekers, this caution might extend to protecting safety, maintaining anonymity, promoting the person's best interests, balancing authentic listening to stories with strategies to prevent vicarious trauma, and engaging in therapist self-disclosure to build trust while maintaining professional boundaries. Taking these considerations into account, occupational therapists might choose to use storytelling as a therapeutic strategy that can support relationship building and contribute to social inclusion of asylum seekers.

Fictional storytelling as a platform for sharing personal stories

The social exclusion of asylum seekers is compounded by their lack of voice due to fears of continued harm if they are identified and found by persecutors, combined with fears of saying something that may jeopardise their chances of obtaining refugee protection from their host country. Fictional storytelling can provide a useful platform for sharing these personal stories. It allows for anonymity and protection for vulnerable storytellers, such as asylum seekers, because identities need not be revealed and sensitive topics that might put the storyteller in danger, or might be difficult to talk about, can be described metaphorically. The occupation of sharing fictional stories can provide voice to asylum seekers within a safe storytelling space.

Fictional folktale storytelling is often considered to be for children. However, this is a remnant of a tradition of 18th and 19th century anthologists censoring complex tales to make them appropriate for young audiences (Chandler, 2012). Folktales can be relevant to people of all ages. In writing the story for this chapter, the author with experience of asylum seeking was a games designer, he was comfortable using the tropes of fiction and particularly science fiction, to tell his stories through metaphors. From a community cultural development perspective, art can provide 'a "container" or safe space for catharsis and the exploration of threatening material' (Marsden, cited in Hunter, 2008, p.7). That said, it is important that the creative product be framed in way that seems age appropriate and personally relevant. Different people have preferences for different forms of storytelling: written, oral, video/televisual, illustrated, sculptural, movement (e.g. dancing and acting), photographic, musical and other story forms across a range of genres (fictional and non-fictional) might be considered depending on the people involved in the storytelling process.

Storytelling can be a useful strategy when working with asylum seekers to create opportunities for self-expression, development of shared understandings, new meanings regarding past experiences, and identifying possibilities for change. Fictional storytelling provides a useful platform for connecting and developing understanding with vulnerable people such as asylum seekers. Ultimately, storytelling can create personal connections and provide substance to calls for more inclusive societies.

This chapter uses fictional storytelling to share the experiences of one asylum seeker (who prefers to remain anonymous, but will sometimes be referred to as the other author), combined with the understandings of two people who are not asylum seekers, based on years of interactions with other asylum seekers. The development of this story involved a dynamic process of co-creation.

The story: Left with nothing but a busted 'delimiter' (and a satchel)

When David first saw the city lights of Targa, they were just a bright smudge on the horizon. He looked at the busted delimiter around his wrist. A crack on the screen was followed by three zeros. He pulled a notebook and pen from his pocket, flipped forward to the latest entry, and read eight, nine, and three zeros - meaning 89,000 points. And then, before doing anything else, before sitting down, before planning how to slip through the city walls unnoticed, even before thinking about Jasmine, he ate an orange. On his wrist, the delimiter clicked forward, to the right of the crack it now read - 005, but he didn't write the new total in his notebook. The taste of the juice in his mouth made him think of his old home. Because, of course, this is not the beginning of the story.

It could begin the day he met Jasmine, singing along to her headphones on a bus, and he offered her an orange just as an excuse to say hello. Or it could start after they jumped over the fire at New Year's and decided to get as many delimiter points as possible; but I don't have to tell you that, you've probably done it yourself, walking every day, enrolling in night classes, adopting a stray cat, drinking mugs of vivi-tea, and all of the sudden you're up 60,000 points. They soon encountered the what-to-do-with-our-points problem, common to so many young relationships. He wanted to book a hiking holiday, she wanted to use the whole lot on a five minute phone call to her grandad in the afterlife.

And so they fought. Mainly about little things. Like what to have for breakfast. Their days fray at the edges. In the end she goes off alone on the hiking holiday she wasn't even sure she wanted.

David was wandering regretfully around his old city and looking at things he wasn't interested in buying when a squirrel popped his head out up from the gutter.

'You're carrying a lot of stuff there.'

Typical squirrel. Thinks David, looking down at his empty hands, they think just because they can talk they have to find something to say at every possible moment. But out loud he says, 'I'm not carrying anything.'

'Oh yes you are. Look at all those thoughts. Mostly about her, and the stuff you did together. Which would be great. If she ever wanted to see you again.'

'She'll see me again. What do you know about it anyway? You're just a squirrel.'

'That makes me an expert in putting things away where they're hard to find.'

'But I don't want to put those memories away. I mean, even if you're right, which you're not, even if she doesn't come back, which she will. I'd still want to be able to think about her.'

'Think about her so much you can't sleep? Think about her so much you wear your shirt back to front?'

David looked down at his shirt and smirked.

'You have to put those thoughts away.' Said the squirrel. 'Trust me on this one.' He dragged over an old brown leather satchel.

'I know what you're thinking. How do you get a memory – something you can't touch – into a bag.' It wasn't easy. After days of visiting the squirrel David managed to get one memory, the easiest possible kind of memory, into the satchel. Nothing significant. Just them waiting in line to buy movie tickets one night in the rain. The feeling of cold water dripping on the back of his neck. That sort of thing. It went in the satchel and was gone. Not as if it had never happened, but it just didn't pop into his thoughts the way it used to – and that made him want more.

Every day he visited the squirrel – and every day he put more memories of Jasmine into the satchel.

He started to worry that if she returned he might not even recognise her – so he decided to ask the squirrel's advice.

But the squirrel had disappeared; and mermaids and mermen were slithering through the canals into the city. Everything changed. At first, people started telling stories about their terrible, mesmerising stare; about not being able to look away. But most people were too busy to care, even when they swam through the fountains outside government house and into the building itself.

'Anyway,' said David's neighbour, Sam, 'the government we had were idiots. Who knows? Maybe these guys will be better.'

At first the changes seemed fairly harmless. They made it compulsory to play cards every Thursday afternoon – but declared it illegal to use the ace. Which wasn't hard, it just took the joy out of playing cards. They fined people, deducting delimiter points, at every opportunity - they hardly had enough points to keep studying, let alone go on holiday. Sam said he was hiding his points by backing them up onto a USB stick.

On the same day the mer-people announced that standing within ten paces of the water was to be made illegal, Sam walked out of his door and didn't come back.

The mer-police came to interrogate David about Sam's whereabouts. David said he had no idea. They charged David with 'playing cards with an ace' and took him away in a van. Before they could get to the police station though, their tails started to dry out so they stopped to get some water from the river – David grabbed his satchel and ran.

He ran and ran and ran. Until he was standing here, at the border, with an orange in his hand. He crept forward as quietly as possible. But a human being can only be so quiet and it wasn't long before the guards from the city of Targa spotted him.

After that, things are blurry. They ask him his name. He remembers that. They sneer at his broken delimiter.

'Five points!' says a tired, sweating guard. 'What kind of person only has five points?'

David shows them the notebook. Tries to explain that there are plenty of points there – that it's only the screen that's broken. But they sneer even more.

It's hard to talk about the things that happen after that. The long days of sitting in empty rooms. Of eating the same salty food day after day. Of not going anywhere. Of knowing there are games behind locked doors which they are not allowed to play – because they supposedly don't have the points to do it. Out of sheer desperation David uses two points to get up three floors. The view is beautiful. But now it looks like there are only three points left on his delimiter. It's hard to keep track of how many points he really has left. He can feel the place draining them away. There are men there who loose their voices arguing with the guards. Who'll do anything just to feel something new. Whenever he can he puts these things in the satchel. But the satchel is getting heavier.

Then comes the day – when for no very clear reason – a guard takes his delimeter away. He wonders if he will ever see it again; but a few minutes later the guard brings it back and, unbelievably, allows him into the city of Targa itself. He walks around in the sunshine and feels his points surging back. Looking down at his delimiter he realises the screen has been replaced. It isn't perfect, probably second hand; but at least the counter is displaying four digits instead of just three. The screen says 1191 points. He wonders how many he really has.

People still laugh at the delimiter's broken screen and complete strangers want to look inside his satchel. Sometimes they carelessly kick it open, the sadness and the horrors are released, and he has to stuff all those things back in again. Running down a sidestreet one day he sees Sam sitting in the gutter.

'Hey!'

David leans forward to embrace and kiss his friend the way they would have done at home. But then he stops. People don't like that here, so instead he steps away and looks at Sam and smiles. Sam half-smiles back, then looks at the ground. He holds out his arm. He has no points left. 'I can't sleep,' he says, 'I can't get things done. I keep tasting all that salt on my tongue and hearing people argue with the guards. I feel nauseous. My head hurts. My mind hurts. My back hurts. I find myself pulling out my own toenails just to numb the pain. Ever since the delimeter zeroed-out, everything feels worse and I can barely move.'

'You can't think about that stuff.' Says David. 'Here. Put it in the satchel.' But Sam sits stiffly, unable to move.

But the story doesn't end there. Because he takes Sam home and shoves a mug of vivi-tea in his hand. Sam takes a sip, his delimiter clicks over to 000 0001. That's all he can manage for now. Then David sits up all night, while Sam finally sleeps, drawing his design for a portable rollercoaster. Something so small you can fold it up and fit it in your pocket. He plans to roll them out as a worldwide boredom buster.

And that's how we leave them. At 4.15 am – David, enthralled by the physics of rollercoasters. Sam, closing his eyes, his limbs heavy, and his mind free from the horrific memories for a moment. Each of them now with points on their delimiters, hope, choice, and possibilities to engage with the world around them.

The next time you see them, maybe you can check how they're going.

Co-creation

The authors

An online-games designer, creative writer, and occupational therapist came together to co-create the story shared in this chapter. Amongst the group one had been an asylum seeker less than three months before the project began (he is now accepted as a refugee by the Australian government), one had worked in storytelling and community cultural development projects with asylum seekers and other socially excluded groups over ten years, and one had worked with asylum seekers in a range of capacities over eight years including as a program coordinator, a volunteer in community development projects, and as a researcher. With the impetus for writing a story for publication in an occupational therapy text, together they created a fictional story that represents their perspectives on the experiences of asylum seekers. The meetings occurred online because the authors did not live in the same city.

Choosing fiction.

'Stories of persecution are personal and private devastations that are often unspoken,' states Kissoon (2010, p.14). During author meetings, The other author, explained that he preferred not to talk about the challenges he faced as an asylum seeker coming to Australia:

> 'I can talk to you about whatever, but the thing is that I am easily able to just forget about it [a lot of what has happened in my past] so there is nothing that [can] make me sad …. to distract your mind to something that you'd like to think about and not to think about something you don't like …. I block it out.'

Fiction was decided upon as the genre for the story by the three authors because it provided a platform for addressing important issues and concepts related to asylum seekers' experiences indirectly. It did not require The other author to share the details of his personal experiences. Throughout the writing process, the authors would often discuss a concept in fictional terms and the conversation would then turn to connections between fictional concepts and real lived experiences. For example, after identifying concepts from the narrative themes in the initial interview, Alex and Emma brought ideas for fictional devices to the meeting including the delimiter. Devices were discussed, changed, and developed by the group over time. Months later, when reviewing the final version of the story, The other author explained, 'it's like the broken delimiter came out of me. It's like an abstract idea from my real life!'

Writing the story.

Alex and Emma enjoy engaging in writing. For them, writing is both a work and leisure occupation. The other author requested not to write words because English is his second language. He wished to engage in a verbal process for storytelling and chapter development. For him, the occupation of storytelling does not involve written language.

The authors initiated a method for writing the story through an interactive dialogical process of co-creation. The process of co-creation involved verbal storytelling by all participants, discussing, writing, and re-telling the story, creating new meanings with each re-telling.

Discussion topics in the initial meeting were guided by concepts from the Occupational Performance History Interview (Kielhofner, 2004) and concepts regarding the orchestration of occupation (Schell et al, 2014). Drawing from these sources, the discussion topics included:

- identifying life roles
- interests and values,
- stories of daily life and routines,
- meaning and purpose held by activities
- perceptions of personal abilities, skills, and control,
- negotiation of time,

- negotiation with others,
- social and physical environments
- adaptability to changes in environments and differing demands of others.

The other author shared his stories as an asylum seeker and the other authors shared their own stories and understandings. The meeting was recorded, transcribed and reviewed.

Narrative threads were identified in the transcription. For example, 'limited activities in detention centres', 'bored', 'a preference not to talk about challenges faced in the past', 'learning', 'government stopping you from doing what you want to do'. These narrative threads are in line with previous research findings (Campbell & Steel, 2015).

At the second meeting, discussion occurred according to the following sequence: narrative threads, links to possible fictional concepts, relating fictional concepts to real-life experiences, and return to the narrative threads. For example, Alex, the creative writer, suggested a fictional device that could represent the thread of 'a preference not to talk about challenges faced in the past', so all those things that you put aside, it's like, they go into a black box.

The other author said, It's more like a bag, where I put all the things from the past

Emma, the occupational therapist, asked if it might be a backpack that he uses to hold all the negative past experiences, to keep his hands free so that he can do other things. He agreed that keeping his negative past experiences in a bag let him 'do things' but that for him, the bag was not a backpack, it was a satchel: more like an old brown bag that goes over your shoulder, and it has a lid that goes over the top

The other author then moved on to having learnt this strategy from a friend in his home country, and perhaps there could be a character in the book that is a teacher and a friend.

Each author re-told parts of the story from their own perspective, and as a group they refined the characters, devices and storyline. The other author, as a games designer, also brought forward the process of world-design and as a group the authors shared their understandings of the world, or environment, in which the main character (representing an asylum seeker) lived.

A transcript of the second recorded meeting was typed and sections of the verbalisations of the content for the chapter were cut and pasted into a document to form the first draft of the story. The story was then re-written to be easier to read and more cohesive by Alex.

Several cycles of re-telling the story, discussion, and adapting the story text occurred until all authors were satisfied with the content and structure of the story. A similar process was followed for the introductory and concluding text for this chapter.

How might occupational therapists use storytelling?

A story holds 'no single truth' (Richardson, 2000, p.934). There are many ways of understanding what a story means and therefore stories offer an open space for sharing, creating meaning, respecting differences, and developing understandings. Through the process of storytelling and listening, occupational therapists might create strong connections with the people they work with, they might foster connections amongst others by supporting storytelling beyond the immediate storytelling environment, and where appropriate, they might use the content of the stories told by their clients to engage in advocacy. Through creating connections or advocating for social change, occupational therapists can contribute to more inclusive societies using storytelling.

Stories also change through re-telling (Clouston, 2003). In the authors' experience, once co-creation began, a flow of stories (real and fictional) began and personal insights became easier to express. The story changed each time it was told. Re-telling and relating as well as co-creation are suggested strategies for occupational therapists to engage in storytelling.

Re-telling and relating

Re-telling of the story and relating personal experiences to the fictional devices, characters, contexts, and storyline can prompt valuable discussions, which might be personally therapeutic or socially transformative. This story might serve as a point for initiating conversations about occupation, about asylum seekers' experiences, and about the experiences of others who experience persecution or discrimination. The conversations might occur with other professionals and with clients (individuals, groups, or communities). For example, consider the questions that are presented below.

*   Can you relate to this story? What parts of the story are familiar to you? What is familiar about them?
*   Is there a squirrel in your life? What have you learnt from your squirrel? What did the squirrel bring to you?
*   What intangible structures or forces in today's society might be represented by the delimiter?
*   Who controls if, how, or when, a person engages in activities that are meaningful in their life? Who has control over a person's delimiter? Who should have control over a person's delimiter?
*   Would you trust someone if they came to you and said their delimiter was broken?
*   How would you feel if your delimiter was broken? What would you do? Who would be able to help you?
*   Do you have a place where you keep past experiences so that you can remain engaged in what is important to you? Is it also a satchel? Is it a different type of bag?
*   Is it an entirely different vessel? With whom would you be happy to show all the contents?
*   Would you believe someone if they came to you and told you about the mermaids?

Co-creation

Engaging in world-design, description and development of characters, creation of devices, identifying storyline, and integrating meaning in stories with clients can allow development of shared understandings of environments, people, and occupations. Co-creation of stories can also shape understandings of past experiences. Appendix 1 provides prompts for story co-creation based on the process used in the development of the story shared in this chapter.

Co-created stories might be fictional or they might be real-life stories. Working with clients to co-create and share their own stories might serve as an individual therapeutic process or as a way of sharing experiences linked to social disadvantage and engaging with broader social issues. Human connections are formed through the process of co-creation. These relationships between therapists and clients, along with the sharing of stories to develop wider community connections and advocate for social change can contribute to more inclusive societies.

References

Andersson, H.E. and Nilsson, S. (2011) Asylum seekers and undocumented migrants' increased social rights in Sweden. *International Migration*, 49, 167-188

Bonsall, A. (2012) An examination of the pairing between narrative and occupational science. *Scandinavian Journal of Occupational Therapy*, 19, 92-103

Burchett, N. and Matheson, R. (2010) The need for belonging: The impact of restrictions on working on the wellbeing of an asylum seeker. Journal *of Occupational Science*, 17, 85-91

Campbell, E.J. and Steel, E.J. (2015) Mental distress and human rights of asylum seekers. *Journal of Public Mental Health*, 14, 1-18

Chandler, R. (Ed.) (2012) *Russian Magic Tales from Pushkin to Platonov.* London: Penguin.

Clouston, T. (2003) Narrative methods: Talk, listening and representation. *British Journal of Occupational Therapy*, 66, 136-142

Connor Schisler, A.M. and Polatajko, H.J. (2002) The individual as mediator of the person, occupation, environment interaction: Learning from the experience of refugees. *Journal of Occupational Science*, 9, 82-92

Field, O. (2006) Alternatives to detention of asylum seekers and refugees. *Legal and Protection Policy Research Series.* United Nations High Commissioner for Refugees

Galheigo, S.M., Oliver, F.C., Gomes, F. and Aoki, M. (2012) People with disabilities and participation: Experiences and challenges of an occupational therapy practice in the city of São Paulo, Brazil. in N. Pollard & D. Sakellariou (Eds.) *Politics of Occupation-Centerefugeered Practice: Reflections on occupational engagement across cultures.* Chichester: Wiley-Blackwell (pp 128-145)

Hunter, M.A. (2008) Cultivating the art of safe space, research in drama education. *Journal of Applied Theatre and Performance*, 13, 5-21

Hynes, P. (2011) *The Dispersal and Social Exclusion of Asylum Seekers: Between liminality and belonging,* Portland: Policy Press

Kalt, A., Hossain, M., Kiss, L. and Zimmerman, C. (2013) Asylum seekers, violence and health: A systematic review of research in high-income host countries. *American Journal of Public Health*, 103, 3, e30-e42

Kielhofner, G. (2004) *A User's Manual for the Occupational Performance History Interview*

(Version 2.1), OPHI-II, Chicago The Model of Human Occupation Clearinghouse, Department of Occupational Therapy, College of Applied Health Sciences, University of Illinois

Kissoon, P. (2010) From persecution to destitution: A snapshot of asylum seekers' housing and settlement experiences in Canada and the United Kingdom. *Journal of Immigrant & Refugee Studies,* 8, 4-31

Mattingly, C. (1998) *Healing Dramas and Clinical Plots: The narrative structure of experience.* Cambridge, UK: Cambridge University Press

Mattingly, M. and Lawlor, C. (2000) Learning from stories: Narrative interviewing in cross-cultural research. *Scandinavian Journal of Occupational Therapy,* 7, 4-14

Morville, A.L., Amris, K., Eklund, M., Danneskiold-Samsøe, B. and Erlandsson, L.K. (2014) A longitudinal study of changes in asylum seekers ability regarding activities of daily living during their stay in the asylum center. *Journal of Immigrant and Minority Health,* 17, 3, 1-8

Morville, A.L. and Erlandsson, L.K. (2013) The experience of occupational deprivation in an asylum centre: The narratives of three men. *Journal of Occupational Science,* 20, 212-223

Polkinghorne, D.E. (1991) Narrative and self-concept. *Journal of Narrative and Life History,* 1, 135-153

Pollard, N. (2012) Communities of writing. In N. Pollard and D. Sakellariou (Eds.) *Politics of Occupation-Centred Practice: Reflections on occupational engagement across cultures.* Chichester: Wiley-Blackwell (pp146-161)

Price, M.E. (2010) *What is 'Persecution'? Rethinking asylum: History, purpose and limits.* Cambridge: Cambridge University Press

Price-Lackey, P. and Cashman, J. (1996) Jenny's story: Reinventing oneself through occupation and narrative configuration. *American Journal of Occupational Therapy,* 50, 306-314

Raveendran, M. (2012) Plight of the boat people: How to determine state obligations to asylum seekers. *Notre Dame Law Review,* 87, 1277-1312

Refugee Claimants Support Service (2006) *Alone Together.* Brisbane, Australia: Queensland University of Technology

Richardson, L. (2000) Writing: A method of inquiry. In N.K. Denzin and Y.S. Lincoln (eds.) *Handbook of Qualitative Research.* 2nd ed. Thousand Oaks, California: Sage Publications

Rosenberger, S. and Konig, A. (2012) Welcoming the unwelcome: The politics of minimum reception standards for asylum seekers in Austria. *Journal of Refugee Studies,* 25, 537-554.

Sakiyama, M., Josephsson, S. and Asaba, E. (2010). What is participation? A story of mental illness, metaphor, and everyday occupation. *Journal of Occupational Science,* 17, 224-230

Scaletti, R. and Hocking, C. (2010) Healing through story telling: An integrated approach for children experiencing grief and loss. *New Zealand Journal of Occupational Therapy,* 57, 66-71

Schell, B.A.B., Gillen, G., Scaffa, M. and Cohn, E.S. (Eds.) (2014). *Willard & Spackman's Occupational Therapy,* Philadelphia: Wolters Kluwer Health/Lippincott Williams & Wilkins.

Steindl, C., Winding, K. and Runge, U. (2008) Occupation and participation in everyday life: Women's experiences of an Austrian refugee camp. *Journal of Occupational Science,* 15, 36-42

Stewart, E. (2008) Exploring the asylum-migration nexus in the context of health professional migration. *Geoforum.* 39, 1, 223-235

Sweet Freedom Ltd. (2015) *Sweet Freedom Projects: Scattered People.* Sweet Freedom Ltd.

[Accessed 28 October 2015 at http://www.sweetfreedom.org.au/scatteredpeople.html]

Tyler, J.A., and Swartz, A.L. (2012). Storytelling and transformative learning. in E. W. Taylor and P. Cranton (Eds.) *The Handbook of Transformative Learning: Theory, research, and practice.* Chichester: Wiley (pp. 455-470)

Westoby, P. and Dowling, G. (2009) *Dialogical Community Development: With depth, hospitality and solidarity,* West End, Queensland: Tafina Press

Whiteford, G. (2011) From occupational deprivation to social inclusion: Retrospective insights. *The British Journal of Occupational Therapy,* 74, 12, 545

World Federation of Occupational Therapy (2011) *Position Statement on Human Rights.* World Federation of Occupational Therapy. [Accessed 6 October 2011 at http://www.wfot.org/office_files/WFOT HR PP with Canadian Enablement Model.pdf]

Wright St Clair, V. (2003) Storymaking and storytelling: Making sense of living with multiple sclerosis. *Journal of Occupational Science,* 10, 46-51

Appendix 1. Story co-creation prompts for occupational therapists.

Aspect of the story	Definition	Storytelling prompts
World-design	Imagining and describing the environment in which the story occurs.	Where does the story happen? When you are there, what can you see? What are the rules in the place where the story happens? How is the place where the story happens the same/ different to where we are now?
Characters	Imagining and describing plays a part in the story. Each person is described.	Who is each character? How old is the character? Is the character male or female? What do they look like? What would you think of them if you met them? Are they like anyone you know (or not like anyone you know)? How? Why is this character important for telling your story/ sharing your message? Who is the main character? Is there anything that happens in the story that needs another character?
Devices	The objects in the story that represent the main ideas. They often have a causal effect. These objects might make the events in the storyline occur.	What are the main ideas in the story? What objects might represent those main ideas? – these could become the devices for the story. What are the aspects/functions of the device? And what ideas do they represent? Does the device make something happen? How does it work? Does the device belong to one of the characters?
Storyline	A list of the set of events that occur in the story. Storylines can be described in terms of what the characters do (occupation) within the world, using or being affected by the devices.	What happens in this story? Who or what makes it happen? How does the story start? How does the reader meet the characters? What happens in the middle? What is the major event/climax/problem? How is this resolved? What happens in the end? Will everything be explained in the end or will the story leave some parts of the story un-told? Will you present the storyline chronologically (as you imagine it occurs over time) or out-of-order (e.g. including memories, flash-backs, or visions of the future)? Does the reader know everything from the beginning? Does the reader need to learn information throughout the story? Will there be any surprises for the reader in the story?

Appendix 1. Story co-creation prompts for occupational therapists (Continued)

Aspect of the story	Definition	Storytelling prompts
Meaning	The significance of the story and its parts.	What does the story mean to you? What might it mean to other people? Are there parts of the story that are more important than others? When you re-read or re-tell the story, does it have the same meaning as the first time you told the story? Who would you like to hear your story?

Chapter 8
The role of design to support meaningful occupation

Paul Chamberlain and Claire Craig

Introduction

Occupational therapy believes in the importance of enabling people to do the occupations that are necessary and important to them and through these to participate in society of which they are a part. However this concern is not unique to occupational therapy but is shared by other disciplines. Design is one such discipline that is concerned with enabling individuals to engage in meaningful activities through products, environments and services. Whilst design and occupational therapy have emerged from separate traditions in many respects the questions and dilemmas they face are very similar. Both designer and therapist ask: how do we find ways to understand the activities that are of value to individuals and groups? how can we develop methods and approaches to engage individuals in meaningful ways and elicit their understanding, particularly when those individuals are regarded as vulnerable or disenfranchised from society?

This chapter describes methods and approaches that can help to address such questions and in doing so to support inclusion and social innovation for older people. We consider how these approaches pioneered by researchers in Lab4Living (www.lab4living.org.uk), an interdisciplinary research group at Sheffield Hallam University, can help to challenge societies current problematisation of ageing. The chapter begins by highlighting some of the challenges facing older people and how societal attitudes can frequently contribute to occupational deprivation (Whiteford, 2000) to the detriment of health and quality of life. Through a series of case studies we will illustrate how older people have been empowered to co-create strategies, products and through engaging in our research to experience meaningful occupation. We end with reflections on the value of these approaches to interdisciplinary working.

The value of occupation

According to the Constitution of the World Health Organisation (1946) health is not the absence of disease but 'a state of complete physical, social and mental well-being'. Health is seen in its widest sense with an emphasis on an individual's personal resources as well as physical capabilities. This reflects well the philosophy of occupational therapy, which is about enabling people to do activities that are necessary and important to them and through these to participate in society of which they are a part. For occupational therapists the concept of meaningful occupation is seen as essential to health and wellbeing (Wilcock, 1998; Yerxa et al., 1990). Meaningful occupation has been shown to promote feelings of belonging and provide social connectedness (Hasselkus, 2011; Hammell, 2004). The activities we participate in contribute to and reinforce our sense of identity (Wright St Clair et al., 2005; Christiansen, 2000) and can offer a sense of purpose leading to feelings of accomplishment (Leufstadius et al., 2008). Engagement in meaningful activities can more practically provide a structure to the day (Hasselkus, 2011; Townsend & Polatajko, 2007) and offer physical and mental stimulation.

If participation in meaningful occupation is so integral to health and wellbeing, the loss or absence of opportunity for engagement has serious ramifications. Occupational deprivation is a term that has been used to describe the absence of or systematic denial of opportunities for individuals to engage in activities that have personal, social or cultural meaning (Hocking & St.Clair, 2011). The causes of occupational deprivation are wide-ranging and include broader political and socio-economic determinants and inequalities as well as individual circumstances which may occur as the consequence of caregiving or the breakdown of family relationships.

Older people can be particularly vulnerable to experiencing occupational deprivation. Increasing physical and cognitive frailty can act as significant barriers to participation in meaningful activity, particularly when this is accompanied by the loss of income and the physical resources to compensate. However equally disabling are societal attitudes, which can problematise ageing. Even though ageing is part of the life-course, older people are generally still viewed through the medical model that focuses on impairment and from a position that reflects the idea that individuals need to be monitored or need help and assistance (Katz et al, 2011).

Older people have therefore tended to be viewed with pity and as passive recipients rather than as active participants in research. It is less common to find research that focuses on the broader aspirations in relation to their lives. Research has revealed how people aged over seventy are persistently seen as incapable and pitiable when compared with other groups and there is unthinking disregard for older people's preferences and aspirations (Dignity in Care, 2012). As one older person recently commented to the authors,

'I tell you what is the worst thing that I come across and it still annoys me now is some people not all people but some people treat you like you're brain dead. And they are so patronizing as if because you're retired your brain's gone. You know they took it out when you left work they took it out and gave it to somebody else. It really annoys me when they do that.'

Researchers and clinicians working with older people need to find ways of challenging these preconceptions. One of the difficulties, however, is that the methods we use to elicit information can frequently reinforce the stereotypes around ageing that currently exist. Older people can be quickly reduced to the information contained on the tick lists and paper based assessments that are often used in health services. These can, at worst, focus only on deficits, or at the very best engage people at a very superficial level. This can be a particular challenge for occupational therapists attempting to capture the richness of a person's occupational identity.

Another issue with this approach is that it creates a fundamental power imbalance. Where such methods are used the researcher or clinician effectively holds the locus of control so that the process involves more of a doing to..., rather than uncovering with... The information elicited can consequently relate more to what the clinician or researcher thinks is important rather than what the person sees as being significant.

> The design of products and of environments in relation to older people can be equally disabling. Many aids and adaptations place perceived function above form and the actual experience of use, with the consequence that the range of products available are limited, so that rather than being seen as desirable possessions they serve rather to reinforce loss and emphasize vulnerability. As Greenhalgh (2013, p.87) writes:, 'medicine is a material culture and technologies contain material features: materiality includes sociological implications of these: digital goods have cultural meaning. Some such as ipads symbolise status independence, modernity and youth; others such as alarms or incontinence detectors may symbolise the opposite cultural phenomena: decay, dependence, stigma and loss of youth.

Again there can be a focus on deficits, feeding into much of the stigma around ageing that currently exists which in turn can further reinforce attitudes, contributing to occupational deprivation and social exclusion. This can be particularly true in relation to the development of technologies for older people, which very much reflect the idea that individuals need to be monitored or need help and assistance.

How can such stereotypes be challenged and how can we find ways to understand the richness of the occupations in people's lives in order to design products, environments and services that will promote human flourishing through engagement in meaningful occupation?

These are questions that a group of researchers have been exploring over the last ten years. Lab4Living is an interdisciplinary research group at Sheffield Hallam University, UK, that brings together designers, occupational therapists, engineers and fine artists. The fundamental philosophy of the lab is to:

> develop environments and propose creative strategies for future living in which people of all ages and abilities not merely survive but are enabled and empowered to live with dignity, independence and fulfillment. (www.lab4living.org)

The underpinning premise is that no one profession holds the answers, but by crossing disciplinary boundaries and drawing on respective strengths, we can engage in acts of collective creativity to develop holistic human centred approaches to address significant societal questions.

These approaches reflect very much the changing role of designers as articulated by Sanders (2003). According to Sanders, through the evolution of human-centered design practices we have seen a shift in focus from individual to collective creativity that has presented a new role for designers as creators of scaffolds or infrastructures upon which non-designers can express their creativity. Bohm (1998) suggested everyone is creative but non-designers are generally not in the habit of expressing their creativity that is likely to be latent. All people have a wellspring of creativity when it comes to experiences they care about, such as home, hobbies etc. but applied less broadly than designers. Sanders suggested the new role of designers will be to learn how to access and understand the aspirations of ordinary people to create scaffolds that help people realize their dreams. 'Designers will transform from being designers of 'stuff' to being the builders of scaffolds for experiencing. And ordinary people will begin to use and express their latent creativity' (Sanders, 2001, p.1).

Lab4Living very much adopts a lifespan approach, recognising that individuals face potential challenges across the life-course. However we have a particular interest in the role of design in promoting wellbeing in older people. Our research in this respect is based on the premise that older people offer a valued resource and asset (through their lived experience) to families, community and society and we have actively sought ways to tap into these strengths. What follows are brief descriptions of three research projects where, through utilising methods of co-creation, older people have been active partners in designing products and environments to maximise occupational engagement and through the process themselves have been empowered. The chapter ends with our reflections of the potential of this approach to enabling and supporting social innovation and inclusion.

Future bathrooms

The first case study we describe is a research project entitled *Future Bathrooms*. We often associate the bathroom with a range of occupations relating to self-care and personal activities of daily living. It is the place where we bathe, where many of the tasks associated with grooming take place but it is easy to forget that having a bath or a shower is not only about keeping clean. For children bath-time can be about play and fun, as we age bathing can be a valued leisure activity, an opportunity to experience relaxation. The bathroom is the place where much grooming, fashioning of hair, applying make-up take place and these are all ways we can express our personality, creating our own unique style. Culturally the act of bathing can be associated with rituals necessary for the expression of faith.

Yet the bathroom is a place full of contradictions. It can be a place of fun and relaxation, of intimacy and privacy but it can also be the room in the house associated with vulnerability and risk. For older people experiencing changes in dexterity, a decline in mobility and loss of visual acuity, bathing can become a chore and concerns about falling can result in the bathroom becoming a place to be feared.

Understanding the needs of older people who use the bathroom and creating environments to facilitate independence and promote continued engagement in the core occupations that take place there, is an important concern for both occupational therapists and designers alike. However, building this understanding is not without its challenges. The bathroom is a space of private and intimate ritual, such as when and how we wash or go to the toilet. Discussion of these intimate acts can be regarded as taboo and traditional research methods such as questionnaires, interviews and observational techniques are potentially too intrusive. Whilst motion capture technology can offer some ergonomic insights regarding how individuals may navigate getting in and out of the bath or on and off a toilet, it cannot record the emotional and sensory aspects of user engagement and interaction.

The aim of the *Future Bathroom* study was to develop a robust methodology for fostering co-design dialogue between designers, researchers and older people. Particular emphasis was placed on individuals who, as a consequence of living with chronic age related health conditions such as arthritis, stroke and macular degeneration, were unable to participate in valued bathing and grooming activities. Rather than designing adaptive equipment, which can sometimes further stigmatise older users and make the bathroom less accessible to the whole family, the study explored whether it was possible to create a space that had the flexibility to evolve and grow to reflect the changing needs of individuals and their families as they age.

Rather than conceptualising design as a problem solving activity used at the end of the development process to embellish a product, we used design and the creation of objects to make tangible concepts and ideas to promote discussion and to aid communication. These critical artefacts and prototypes became key to the research as they aided participants in accessing their tacit knowledge, by demonstrating the things they did through doing, rather than trying to verbalise the things they did intuitively.

Our research approach was underpinned by the principle of designing with people rather than designing for people. We recognised that the way a young designer might think about the bathroom space would be very different to how an older person may conceptualise this. To enable the project team to develop rich insights into older people and bathroom use, a group of older people were recruited to the project and trained as community researchers, becoming employees of the university. The community researchers undertook a series of home visits. Equipped with a researcher pack comprising of a camera, note-book, and prompt cards, these community researchers interviewed dependent and independent older residents, recording their bathroom facilities through photographs and drawings. The community researchers were able to empathise and gather more intimate stories than would have emerged through more traditional research methods or if the younger academic research team had conducted the visits.

Following the visits a series of co-design workshops bringing together the researchers and designers were held (fig 1). Here people engaged in the production of objects, tangible manifestations of discussions and visions of potential bathroom products for the future (Chamberlain et el, 2012).

Fig 1. *Future bathroom*: Co-designing with users

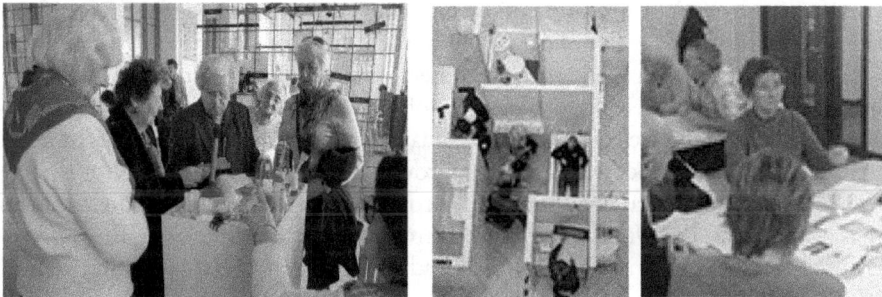

The outcome of the project met its aim to foster a co-design dialogue and resulted in the development of methods to support the creation of a community of older people who were engaged in imaginative activities, mutual problem solving, embracing risk and innovative ideas. Emerging ideas continue to be developed with manufacturers for potential mainstream commercial application rather than as specialist products. However, more than this, the process itself had offered a valued occupation for many individuals who were engaged in research, a form of employment and confidence. As well as ideas and design solutions for potential products that emerged from the project, there was recognition of the value of learning that had taken place, was included in the Department of Health (2011) Parliamentary report on Research and Development Work Relating to Assistive Technology (2010-11), and prompted the development of a booklet, endorsed by Age UK (www.Lab4living.org.uk). Engagement in the project empowered the community researchers and as informed participants they are able to better support their own actions and decision making as well support and advise others as experts.

Engagingaging: Stigmas

Future bathrooms underlined the value of designing with people and the potential use of objects, of critical artefacts to scaffold ideas and maximise engagement. However as the participants we worked with highlighted, older people can be disabled far more as a consequence of societal attitudes to ageing than by poorly designed environments. The design of desirable objects which maximise independence but at the same time do not label or stigmatise older people can help to address some of these preconceptions and promote social inclusion. However, if we are truly to promote occupational engagement we need to challenge some of these deeply held societal stereotypes. Our second case study, a transnational research platform entitled *Engagingaging* sought to do just this.

The research aimed to understand the needs of the ageing population to inform the design of products and systems to support independence and wellbeing in later life. Our focus was a comparison of the experiences of older people living in Taiwan with those of older people in the United Kingdom. Taiwan was selected for study as it has a comparable landmass with the UK (small island), and it has a fast developing high-tech industry with one of the world's highest concentration of Internet access. Its traditional culture where older children look after elderly parents is changing, many moving to work overseas, and like many countries it is experiencing a significant demographic shift as a result of an ageing population

In collaboration with academic researchers at Chang Gung University's Product Design Research lab we conducted a series of workshops and home visits with older people in their respective countries. Initial data were captured using semi structured interviews but with a focused discussion around objects. Participants from the UK were recruited from local care homes and community groups e.g. Sheffield Elders, Sheffield 50+ and the University of the Third Age. Participants from Taiwan were recruited from the Chang Gung Health and Cultural Village, a vast purpose built community (4,500 residents) for older people. This was complimented by home visits in the UK and Taiwan to engage with people living independently (Chamberlain &

Craig, 2013).

Again, the philosophical drive for our multi-method approach to engagement was researching with rather than on older people, who were positioned as active participants rather than passive respondents. Collective creativity as described by Saunders (2003) was again the vehicle, and whilst our focus was on older people we embraced a far broader demographic. However, in co-design products are often not designed by the users themselves, but they contend, and move on to outline a set of principles that can be designed into an artefact in order to transfer design capability to the users (Von Hippel & Katz, 2002).

Using a practice-based research methodology (www3.shu.ac.uk/c3ri/adit/) we developed the equivalent of a grounded theory approach, transforming data collected through these interviews into objects, in this instance, pieces of furniture. The collection of furniture was entitled *Stigmas* (fig 2) created by Chamberlain to embody the experiences shared and informed by older people of the physical and attitudinal challenges they faced in everyday life. The objects, conceptualised, as critical artifacts, were not presented as solutions but as vehicles through which to engage people, promote discussion, raise questions, challenge preconceptions, and generate more in-depth data. Ultimately we sought to further not just our understanding but also the understanding of all those who engaged with them.

Fig 2. Stigmas

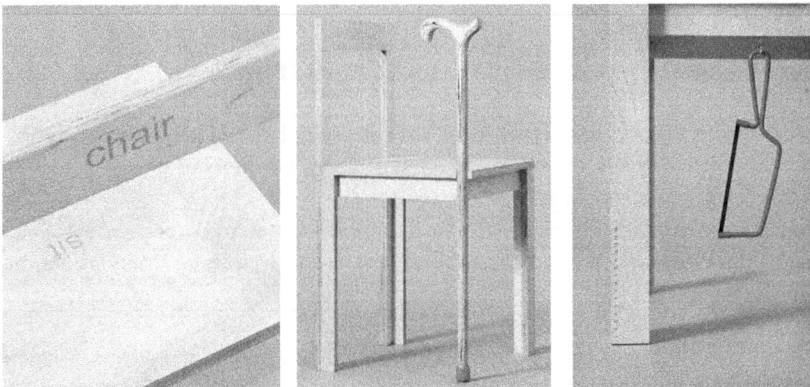

A selection from the Stigmas series – right to left -- 'This is a chair to sit on', 'Rest of your life', 'Adjustable chair'. Critical artefacts, part of the engagingaging platform that present a landscape of later life, posing questions not answers.

Rather than reinforcing a medicalised view of ageing by exhibiting the work in hospitals and care settings, the works were shown in a number of highly prestigious galleries, including the Museum of Contemporary Art, Taipei, the Building Centre, London, the Taipei Cultural Centre and the SIA gallery Sheffield.

The scale of this was immense; the Museum of Contemporary Art in Taipei was housed within the Underground metro station, which saw a footfall of over forty five thousand people a week. Linked to each of the exhibitions was a series of workshops that included older people, families, design students, health students, medical professionals and the Chinese community (Sheffield, UK) where people were asked to consider and make a model of their dream space. The research and photographs of the exhibition appeared on the front of the China Post newspaper with one of the World's largest readerships.

Chamberlain has described how the concept of the exhibition is embedded within the culture of art and design and has a long history as a form of gathering employed to prompt academic discourse. The period (17th century) in which these salons dominated has been labeled the 'age of conversation' and salons themselves 'theatres of conversation' (Chamberlain & Craig, 2013). Throughout the exhibitions and workshops the debate the research generated was enormous. Audiences viewing the exhibition spoke of seeing projections of their future-selves in the exhibits. The curator of the Museum of Contemporary Art in Taipei summed this up when he said:

Figure 3. Engagingaging

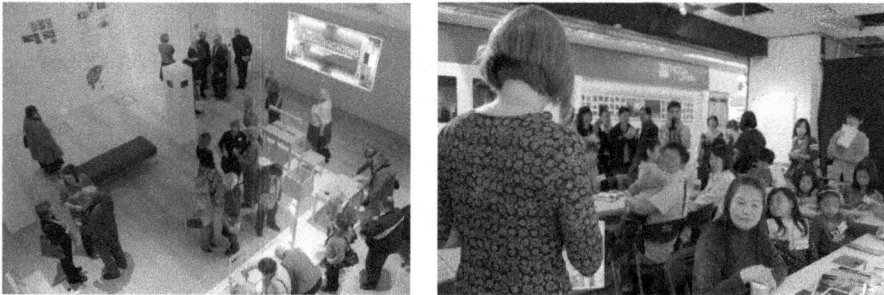

Theatre for conversation -- was a transnational research platform utilising exhibition as a research tool provided a forum to engage with large numbers of people across continents to explore issues of ageing.

'The artifacts in the exhibition stimulate deep thought related to older people for participants and visitors. It announces and informs the awareness of issues we might all face in the future.'

Questions emerged through the workshops regarding our conceptions of ageing and the discussion was enriched because of the cross-cultural exploration of this. There was a detailed exploration of dream spaces and the role of the environment in promoting or inhibiting valued roles and meaningful activity (research.shu.ac.uk/.../engagingaging-exhibition-at-moca-studio-taipei).

The research itself reaffirmed the importance of meaningful occupation throughout the life-course. A sense of community emerged as an important theme. Many positive responses emerged from those who participated in communal activities, e.g. game clubs, bridge (UK), Mah-Jong (TW) singing groups, physical activity, Tai Chi (TW) and walking groups (UK). A structure and sense of place was important to facilitate such activities, however the ability for individuals to choose to participate in such activities was crucial.

The importance for older people to maintain cultural and intellectual life, through music, cooking, art and craft was also re-affirmed. There was an acknowledgement within the research findings that the need for older people to keep learning must be tempered with recognition that older people have a valued role in sharing and passing on their valuable experiences. The importance of continuing to make a contribution to society and feeling valued is significant and many participants engaged in volunteer work.

Older people participating in the workshops spoke of the importance of having a voice. One person articulated this in the following way: 'I am so glad someone is thinking about us and the exhibition is a great opportunity for us to share our experiences with younger people.'

Many pre-conceptions were challenged, particularly in relation to the views of many of the younger researcher's about older people's use of technology. Generally younger participants collectively took the position that older people struggle with all types of new technology and specifically design students felt that it was their role to make products easier to use for older people. However the workshops revealed many adept older users of technology and a variety of reasons why older users might not extensively interact with technology. Often it was not the case they could not but they either did not see a need to or could not be bothered.

Objects and critical artefacts offered valuable ways to begin to understand the richness of occupation in people's lives. The Exhibition created the conduit, through which societal assumptions relating to ageing could be made visible, explored and to some degree challenged. The exhibition was a meeting space that enabled this to happen.

However we were mindful that whilst we had engaged with a significant number of people, those individuals who were exceptionally frail, particularly marginalised and unable to access the exhibition could in some way be excluded from these conversations. The third case study therefore describes how we translated the principles of the exhibition into a format that could be viewed within a person's own home.

Exhibition in a box

Exhibition in a box explored the experiences of older people across Europe to build understanding of how design can support independence and wellbeing in later life. The research built on methods developed within *engagingaging* and central to this was the notion of exhibition as a research tool. However rather than the onus being placed on older people to physically access a traditional exhibition space, *exhibition in a box* (fig 4) distilled the essence of the exhibition into a suitcase which could be transported to the person's home. In doing so the home was transformed into the research arena, providing individuals with a tangible prompt to scaffold conversation.

Twelve boxes were produced and distributed for use with health specialists in collaboration with older users across Europe. These boxes comprised of everyday objects, photographs and textual material defined through the user-workshops undertaken in conjunction with the earlier large-scale exhibitions in *engagingaging*.

The objects were carefully selected to code, represent and prompt further discussion on themes that had emerged from the earlier research. Key themes included mobility, hygiene, relationships, identity, communication, technology, food, art, money, recreation, safety and work and these were represented through the set of found objects that included, keys, dice, soap, pencil, watch, stone, glove, post-card, spoon. The objects could and did combine to create objective correlatives prompting and enabling participants to express emotional responses. For example, pencil and post card prompted discussion around travel, communication, technology (analogue vs digital). Each box contained a guide intended to help participants navigate their way around the box, but we deliberately chose not to include anything more prescriptive, seeking to understand how individuals engaged with and made sense of the space. Our approach was to work in partnership with older people, to develop a set of principles that primarily positioned the older person as the expert and encourages choice and decision-making, which we shared with the researchers.

Figure 4: Exhibition in a box

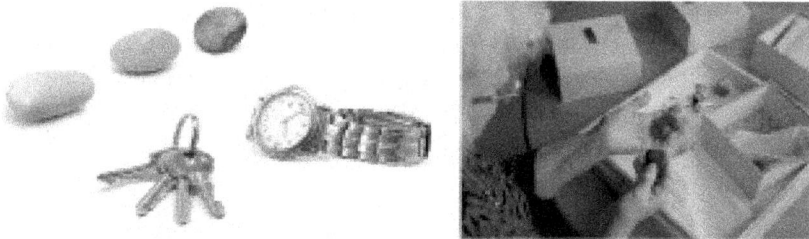

Exhibition distilled into a box. Objects prompting meaningful insights into daily life.

Within the first phase of the research we identified and worked with four occupational therapy departments in Universities across Europe including the Hogeschool Zuyd in the Netherlands and the Zhaw Institute in Zurich. Staff and students under supervision used the methods developed (Chamberlain & Craig, 2013) by the research team and worked with older people in a number of settings. Initial feedback from the workshops to date suggests the *exhibition in a box* facilitates empowerment for older people, providing them with a voice and opportunity for choice and decision-making. The objects have allowed different ways for participants to express their personal identity and in many cases their creativity, prompting them to describe things they have made previously in their life and suggest new ways of doing things. The findings to date also challenge negative assumptions about frail older people and their willingness to participate in activities, which could enhance their own lives and those of others. For example one 70+ year old participant learnt to drive to prove a point to his grandchildren and another 70+ year old who undertook a high wire challenge to raise money for charity.

The real strength of the box is that the objects are something to which everyone can relate, no matter what the culture, language or age of participants. The box speaks something of the universal nature of the tools through which we perform meaningful occupations, offering a point of contact and a way we can gain entry into understanding the value of these things in people's lives. Whilst the objects in the box remain unchanging, the associations they prompt and the stories they evoke are ever changing. Whilst the *exhibition in a box* captures the essence of the larger gallery exhibition, in the context of each person's home it takes on, responds to the components of the environments in which it is examined and in doing so becomes an exhibition in its own right. As a consequence each exhibition is unique because of the iterative and evolving contribution of the participants.

Exhibition in a box has more recently been utilized as a critical artifact methodology by the authors to build understanding of end-users attitudes to technology in everyday life and how it might most appropriately be adopted to support their personal healthcare. The aim is to engage people who are frequently under-represented in telehealth/telecare research by virtue of their age, ethnicity or socio-economic status, in meaningful ways.

Reflections

As stated at the start of this chapter design, like occupational therapy, is about enabling people to do activities that are necessary and important to them and through these to participate in society of which they are a part. Traditionally design does this by being employed in the development of products to positively aid people in their everyday activities. User-centred design is a methodology frequently adopted by designers that focuses on user need to establish understanding to inform the physical designed outcome. However designers also have to be mindful of the technological and economical restraints frequently imposed by the manufacturer (paying client). Balancing these demands is the skill of the designer and success is usually judged on the commercial success of the product outcome. The knowledge emerging from the research could be used as a catalyst or tool to inform development of new commercial ideas. However, as demonstrated by the case studies described in this chapter, design can also be employed to engage people in research and meaningful occupation where the objective is not primarily the creation of a physical commercial product.

At the beginning of this chapter we highlighted how older people can be stigmatised and regarded as vulnerable or disenfranchised as a consequence of societal attitudes. We asked the question, how can such stereotypes be challenged and how can we find ways to understand the richness of the occupations in people's lives in order to design products, environments and services that will promote human flourishing through engagement in meaningful occupation?

The case studies described demonstrate how utilising creative methods through design can facilitate the engagement of people as active partners in research and design activity rather than passive respondents. Formal recognition of people's role as true co-researchers in our projects, *future bathrooms* for example, and utilisation of creative tools, have challenged the power imbalance often created by the academic researcher and research participant (Chamberlain et el, 2012). The Lab4Living team has thoughtfully considered the meeting space, context and environment, to conduct the research. Exhibition formats used extensively within the *future bathroom* and *engagingaging* projects while the home itself becomes the space for the *exhibition in a box*. This has allowed for a more inclusive approach to collaborating with marginalized individuals and communities where they can engage in activities within more familiar and accessible territory. Our approach has empowered individuals providing them with a voice and ability for choice and decision-making enabling them to discuss and undertake activities that are important to them.

The use of carefully selected objects and photographs described through the *exhibition in the box* case study, the prototypes utilised in *engagingaging* and prototypes in *future bathrooms* demonstrate the value of design when employed through objects as critical artefacts. These creative tools can be utilised as vehicles to prompt discussion and enhance communication and each case study highlights how the creative use of design can overcome potential barriers for engagement and collaboration with people such as language, culture, gender and age.

Lab4Living has continued to build a significant community of willing volunteers established through an extensive network of community groups and the diversity of ongoing projects have nurtured a sense of purpose, belonging and social connectedness for the participants. We believe that critical to the success of Lab4Living has been its openness and encouragement in support of interdisciplinary collaboration. This has challenged traditional domain specific approaches and protocols, drawing on and recognising individual strengths to creatively and collectively support new ways of thinking and working.

Individuals and communities actively engaged in our work have been empowered through the process itself, a number of the *future bathroom* participants for example stating how they have been empowered as more informed consumers. The projects have provided opportunity for occupational engagement through meaningful activities, mental and physical stimulation, and in many cases provided a structure to lives of the participants. Our collaborative aim to enhance quality of life for people provides a sense of purpose and accomplishment.

Designers traditionally create objects and through engagement with these individuals can experience meaningful occupation. However the case studies described in this chapter demonstrate how meaningful occupation can also be achieved through the employment of design where individuals are thoughtfully and creatively engaged in the process itself. Our approach has and continues to be applied in a broad range of design led research projects undertaken within Lab4Living (www. Lab4living.org.uk) and we continue to seek and engage new and diverse communities to help us extend our work. However many volunteers continue their long association extending and sharing their expertise.

References

Bohm, D. (1998) *On Creativity*. London: Routledge

Chamberlain, P. and Yoxall, A. (2012) Of mice and men: The role of interactive exhibitions as research tools for inclusive design. *The Design Journal*, 15, 1, 57-78

Chamberlain, P. and Craig, C. (2013) Human-computer interaction. Human-centred design approaches, methods, tools, and environments, Volume 8004 of the series *Lecture Notes in Computer Science*, 22-31

Christiansen, C. (2000) Identity, personal projects and happiness: Self-construction in everyday action. *Journal of Occupational Science*, 7, 98-107

Department of Health (2011) *Parliamentary Report on Research and Development Work Relating To Assistive Technology (2010-11)*. [Accessed 7 March 2016 at https://www.gov.uk/government/uploads/system/uploads/attachment_data/file/215543/dh_127996.pdf]

Dignity in Care (2012) *Delivering Dignity: Securing dignity in care for older people in hospitals and care homes*. London: Dignity in Care.

Greenhalgh, T., Wherton, J., Sugarhood, P., Hinder, S., Practer R. N. and Stones, R (2013) What matters to older people with assisted living needs? A phenomenological analysis of the use and non-use of telehealth and telecare. *Social Science and Medicine*, 93, 86-94.

Hammell, K. W. (2004) Dimensions of meaning in occupations of daily life. *Canadian Journal of Occupational Therapy*, 71, 296-305

Hasselkus, B. (2011) *The meaning of everyday occupation*. (2nd ed). Thorofare NJ; Slack

Hocking, C. and St. Clair, V. W.(2011) Occupational science: Adding value to occupational therapy. *New Zealand Journal of Occupational Therapy*, 58, 1, 29-35

Katz, J., Holland, C., Peace, S. and Taylor, E. (2011) *A Better Life: What older people with high sup- port needs value*. Milton Keynes: Open University.

Leufstadius,C., Erlandsson, L.K., Bjorkman, T and Eklund, M. (2008) Meaningfulness in daily occupations among individuals with persistent mental illness. *Journal of Occupational Science*, 15, 1, 27-35

Sanders, L, (2001) Collective creativity. *AIGA Journal of Interaction Design Education*, 3, 1-6

Sanders, L. (2003) Collective creativity. *AIGA Journal of Interaction Design Education*, 7

Townsend, E.A. and Polatajko, H.J. (2007). *Enabling Occupation II*. Ottawa:CAOT publications.

Von Hippel, E., and Katz, R. (2002) *Shifting Innovation to Users Via Toolkits*. Rochester: Social Science Research Network

Whiteford, G. (2000) Occupational deprivation: Global challenge in the new millenium. *British Journal of Occupational Therapy*, 63, 5, 200-204

Wilcock, A. (1998) A theory of human need for occupation. *Journal of Occupational Science*. 1, 1, 17 -24

Wright St Clair, V., Hocking, C., Bunrayong, W., Vittayakorn, S. and Rattakorn, P. (2005) Older New Zealand women doing the work of Christmas: A recipe for identity formation. *Sociological Review*, 53, 2, 332-350

Chapter 9
The client council: From great movement and little power to little movement and great power

Marijke Burger

Before I got mentally ill I worked as a behavioral therapist (video-interaction model), with people with severe mental illness, retardation and epilepsy. I used the Structural Analysis of Social Behaviour (SASB) (Benjamin,1996), as a means to understand all kinds of behavior. After that I spent some years as chairwoman of the works council of a mental health facility (ambulant care), while working as a coordinator. When I was 41, episodes of bipolar disorder made work impossible. I decided to spend my time contributing to a client council. This was interesting because this was, compared to my previous work in the works council, a totally other point of view on the same matter (mental health issues). I learned that patients are the task of the institution but easily overseen. In the nine years I spent on the client council I became more and more intrigued by the sheer complexity of the task of client councils. This led to the research which is the subject of this chapter. To my knowledge this is the first study on this scale, on this topic, entirely from the point of view of clients.

Introduction

Participation in organizational decision making in health organizations is seen as a basic human right (Commissie van der Burg, 1977) and a reflection of the democratic processes inherent in the Dutch culture. An organization is 'stupid if it fulfills its tasks without the viewpoint of their clients as key-stakeholders', as one of the CEOs (involved in this research project) said. Rights for patients are seen as a line of defense against humiliation and being diminished. Clients must have a say in decisions about their life. The client council law, the Wet Medezeggenschap Cliënten zorginstellingen (WMCZ), the co-determination law for clients in health organizations in effect between the years 1996-2020, stems from this line of thinking. The initial goals of the WMCZ were supposed to strengthen the legal position of the clients on a collective level and to improve the match between the supply and the demand of care.

This chapter, which is based on our research, can be read as a response to the quite frustrating task of giving effect to both goals of this law, the second of which appeared to be especially unfeasible and unrealistic. In 2020, 3 years after our research-report (2017, Clientenraadsels) was published, the new law, named WMCZ 2018 went into effect. This law contained a new article which made the genuine participation of clients mandatory (article 2). To our delight the outcomes of our research are recommended and even included in the nationwide used application which supports the practice of this new law (guideline WMCZ 2018, p9.)

In a lecture about client councils Trappenburg (2004, p.2) raises the question why the client perspective actually should be enforced in the first place:

'Clients and professionals are not enemies (...) nevertheless professionals don't always succeed in taking the perspective of the client into account, (therefore) it is sensible to apply explicit attention to the perspective of clients.'

Client councils are an instrument by which collective legal rights for all clients are established. A client council is a body of about 7 to13 clients with, in this case, mental health problems, which supports, advises and advocates to further the interests of all clients of the organization at management and organizational levels. The client council delivers input into the policy of the organization from a client perspective, with the aim of realizing good quality services that match the clients' wishes.

Enabled by the WMCZ-laws, the client council is also supposed to be an active and tough partner, being a third party next to the management board and the supervisory board in the day to day policymaking structure of the organization. Therefore the client council plays a role in the internal checks and balances of semi-public organizations.

The rights of the client council: Common interests

The client council has several rights: the right to receive the information it needs to fulfill its task; the right to have regular consultations with the management of the organization; the right to give advice (whether it is asked for or not); and the right to ask a court of law to investigate where they suspect mismanagement. Issues of disagreement can be submitted to the (Landelijke) Commissie van Vertrouwenslieden (LCvV) (Committee of Trusted Persons).

The 1996 WMCZ Act made three sorts of advice possible: ordinary advice (regarding systems), strengthened advice (regarding the lifeworld experience of clients) and un-solicited advice (regarding initiatives of the client council).

The service provider is obliged to ask the client council's (strengthened) advice in relation to a number of topics that are stipulated in the Act, for instance, direct client-related issues, nutrition policy in clinics, hygiene, safety policy, spiritual help, recreational facilities, social help, settlements concerning the right to complaint and the appointment of heads of clinics.

There is also an obligation for the service provider to ask the client council (ordinary) advice about organizational changes, changes in the activities of the organization, financial accounts, monitoring and/or improvement of the quality of care systems and the safety systems. This advice has to be asked for at a point in time where the input of the client council can still be taken into account in the decision making process. The council could not meaningfully participate in processes if they are not fully aware of them and therefore they have also to be adequately informed (with the right information in a timely way). The new WMCZ 2018 offers a sharp turn regarding to the focus-change, to empower client councils and clients (who are admitted into mental health facilities).

Difficulties of co-determination by clients in mental health services

The counterbalancing influence on policy structures of semi-public organization by client councils is, and has always been, very much promoted by the government of the Netherlands. The Netherlands Scientific Council for Government Policy (WRR, 2014, p.8) states:

'Client councils do not usually take their role to the extent they are supposed to. The client council as third party does not challenge the other parties sufficiently. This is due to the enormous inequality between the client council and the management board.'

Extended use of the law is quite rare (four to seven cases a year), as can be seen in the archives of the LCvV (National Committee of Trusted Persons), especially in the case of client councils in mental health facilities (Archive LCvV, 2014). Stress-avoidance and difficulty in acting with a united front as a client council are reasons for this. Client councils have limited influence on decision making at policy level. They are merely used as a sounding board. The task of the client council is to influence the policy of the organization, in practice this is very difficult. Our research shows that this task needs reconsidering.

Limitations of the WMCZ law (the co-determination law for clients in health organizations)

During its period as a bill, as well as after it became law in 1996, there was a lot of criticism of the WMCZ. A very thorough assessment of the WMCZ by van der Voet (2005, p. 403), led to the conclusion that most criticism of the WMCZ was well-founded:

'Although a legal prescription for clients' participation appears to be necessary, the form of participation that is prescribed by the WMCZ – that of co-determination through a clients' council – does not in any case appear to be an effective and efficient way to achieve the goals of the WMCZ, i.e. strengthening the legal position of the clients on a collective level and improving the match between the supply and the demand of care...The legislator also did not succeed in finding the right balance in the WMCZ between the things that need to be regulated by law and the things that can be left to self-regulation.'

Client councils (in mental health services) are inherently bureaucratic because there is the law to act upon. Client council's work was merely symbolic because the 1996 WMCZ failed to guarantee the independence of the client council towards the board of the health care organization. Client councils in the mental health area can be fragile too, because the members can be fragile. The 1996 WMCZ law applied to situations characterized by conflicts of interests and inequality of power and asked in fact for great toughness. Often there were difficulties in maintaining continuity. Matters of independence and representativeness were very often questioned.

The costs of these client councils also appeared to be relatively high compared with the costs of other forms of participation. All of these elements existed because the articles in the 1996 WMCZ were unclear on several points. The 1996 WMCZ for example did not answer the question regarding how a representative client council should be put together. Issues included: bureaucracy, inequality, problems of dependence, dis-continuity, symbolic and high costs.

The 1996 WMCZ and the client councils model drew a lot of attention and partly prevented the conceptualization and development of other more direct forms of co-determination, and other forms were rare.

The law was discussed in Dutch parliament (the second Chamber of the States General) throughout the past 20 years. The history of the law showed a good deal of lip-service about improving the position of client councils but up to 2020 no essential changes were made. In May 2015 client councils were invited to inform the members of the parliament about their criticism of the law (Heuts, 2015). Researchers from our team contributed directly to this discussion.

The 'Clientenraadsels' study: Does the client council still have a reason to exist?

This section describes how a team of council members and researchers, who are service-users as well, undertook a three-year qualitative scientific study between 2012-2015 on behalf of the client council of GGZinGeest (a mental health service provider) in the region of Amsterdam, in the Netherlands.

During the years 2009-2012, when reductive government policies in mental health institutions and services increased, the work of the client councils turned out to be meaningless and pointless. Being involved in advice procedures that were tokenistic was harmful to the client council's sense of dignity. It raised the question of the right to exist and it seemed sensible to find alternative ways for collective client influence.

The aim of the research project was to develop a structure and a method of co-determination that would be able to bring about the real, concrete, specific influence of clients in institutions that provide mental health services. While working at this purpose the team became particularly fascinated by the question of what the most efficient type of co-determination of clients could be.

Research questions

The central questions of the research were:
1. What is the essence of co-determination by client councils, according to the different stakeholders?
2. Which approaches can be developed in order to strengthen this essence?

The research team wanted to learn about the ways in which the work of the client council was perceived by their various participants and stakeholders (members of client councils, clients, managers and CEOs). The researchers aimed to identify the claims, concerns and issues according to the following questions:

1. What perceptions exist about client participation by client councils in Dutch mental health care?
2. What expectations and conditions exist with regard to client participation by client councils?
3. What is, according to the stakeholders, the raison d'être of the client council?
4. What are the perceptions of the future of client councils?

Research process

The research was almost entirely performed by service users. It was supported by staff members of the research department of GGZinGeest. The study was shaped in a constructivist mode and therefore the fourth generation evaluation (FGE) model outlined by Guba and Lincoln (1989) was used. This model is termed 'responsive constructivist' as it exemplified a responsive approach by negotiating the parameters and boundaries of the study through an interactive process involving all stakeholders.

Data collection was performed from a range of sources, primarily in GGZinGeest and also in 17 comparable organizations in virtually all parts of the Netherlands, a total of 75 interviews were conducted (see Table 1).

Table 1
Interviews undertaken (n=75)

	GGZinGeest, mental health organization	17 other, similar mental health organizations*
CEO	3	1
Managers	17	7
Staff members client council	3	8
Clients	18	
Members of client councils	16	2
	57	18

*In the Netherlands 17 mental health institutions are similar to GGZ in Geest.

Methods

The methods employed for gathering information included key informant interviews with stakeholders of co-determination (clients, client councils, boards of directors, management), audiotaped meetings of virtually all client council meetings (4 times a month), meetings with CEOs and managers (2 times a month), meetings transferring information and issues according to the research (5), seminars regarding the subject of client councils (8), meeting with a member of parliament (1), focus-group meetings (13), issue/controversy meeting (1), expert meetings (2). A literature study and document review was also carried out. The collection of the data took place between 2012 and 2015.

Arrangements were made regarding conditions for the use of the information. These included no use without permission and informed consent.

Analytic approach

Interviews with stakeholders: Analyzing the data gained in the interviews appeared to be a very intricate process. The analysis involved organizing the data, working with the data, breaking them into manageable units, and searching for patterns. So it took a long time to reduce the data into concepts and the concepts into one core concept. The core concept was a major discovery about what had to be learned. This led to the review of a substantial part of the data from the point of view of this core concept, and, eventually, to creating new approaches to client participation.

This systematic searching and arranging of the interview transcripts was supported by the computer programme Atlas Ti. (http://csscr.washington.edu/papers/14-01. pdf). Atlas.ti is a qualitative data analysis software package (QDA) that can code a number of different media types, and they did facilitate the process. It was great for managing large, complex data sets, coding a lot of text with ease, conducting searches and visualizations in the qualitative data, and discovering, testing and describing patterns and themes in the data.

The audiotaped client council meetings, meetings transferring information and issues according to the research and seminars regarding the subject of client councils, were partly transcribed. Because of the immediate application of the data the client councils encountered a learning process, with lots of experiments and try-outs.

The audiotaped focus-group meetings, issue/controversy meeting and expert meetings were all transcribed and used to confront the evolving ideas with the reality of the stakeholders of the client council.

Meetings with CEOs and managers were approached with the help of the Structural Analysis of Social Behavior (SASB). The SASB is a method of analyzing and studying many different types of social interactions (http://lornasmithbenjamin. com/sasb/). SASB is a natural, biological model that describes social interactions in terms of three different types of interpersonal focus (see Figure 1). Attentional focus (shown by separate surfaces of the model) is the first issue to solve: Is this about you (I focus on other) or is this about me (what shall I do). Each type of focus is described by two dimensions: Affiliation on the horizontal axis (is this friendly or hostile), and Interdependence on the vertical axis (are we sharing space or separating?). Everything interactive is described in terms of these underlying 'primitive basics'. The third type of focus describes what happens when the self actively does to the self what others have done to him/her (treat yourself as you have been treated). Again, possibilities include components ranging from (self) hate to (self) love on the horizontal axis and from (self) control to letting go (of self) on the vertical axis. These two dimensions are plotted along two lines at right angles to one another (i.e., orthogonally) thereby producing a graph divided into four quadrants (created by the intersecting lines representing these two dimensions).

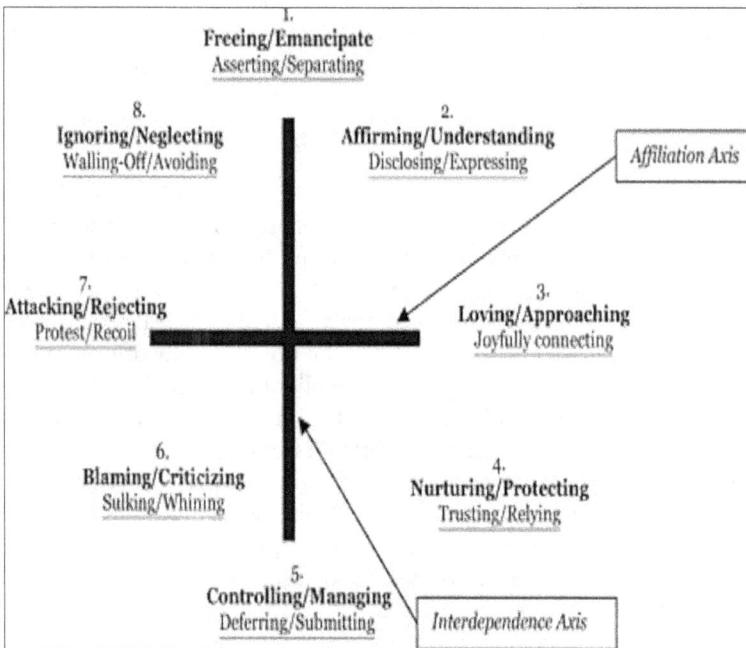

Figure 1:
SASB simplified cluster model. With permission from Prof Elizabeth Skowron, at https://www.researchgate.net/profile/Elizabeth_Skowron/publication/261610712/figure/fig1/AS:267406652211206@1440766122429/Figure-1-SASB-simplified-cluster-model-The-affiliation-axis-is-the-x-axis-and-the.png

Application of the SASB method was particularly interesting in meetings where the client council had to stand up to its rights in order to fulfill its task (power-processes). Exploring the processes on the micro-level brought interesting patterns about group process - loss, submission and power - into light. It played a role in the discovery of sensitizing concepts, it inspired reflection and the combining of ideas. With the help of SASB we saw in the meetings, particularly with the CEOs, some interesting patterns occur: The client council tended on many occasions to self-sabotage, by undermining its own goals. Also forms of self-handicapping were often seen in the material. By being a client council they were, so it seemed, provided with a potential excuse for poor performance. It was also very hard for the members of client council to think beyond themselves, or, on the other hand, to fight for personal issues and make them politic. Themes were found between the axes, where they often remain vague; The dynamic beneath the interactions was that the CEO'S were almost begging for criticism while the client council was afraid to produce this.

Findings from the interviews

The findings answered the central questions of the research.

1. *What is the essence of co-determination by client councils, according to the different stakeholders?*
   All stakeholders were unanimous in their belief that, in order to improve the match between the supply and the demand of care, *the transfer of information* about how clients experience the services is the essence of co-determination. They also foresaw a future in which the perspective of clients in the entire organization is self-evident to such a degree that the client council will not be seen as needed anymore.
2. *Which approaches can be developed in order to strengthen this essence?*
   Researchers and member/experts took some time to create and try out some approaches. All this work led to the next starting points:

   - The relation between professional and client is the place where quality of care originates and can be improved.
   - A great effort has to be made to place the initiative for improvement in the hands of the client.
   - Make it possible for the patient to have an active role in treatment and be confident to give feedback on the quality of it.
   - Make it possible to maximize influence for clients 'on the spot' (during treatment) and also around the spot (the treatment supporting systems).
   - It is not possible to represent people if you have not talked to them. The client council should avoid being in the position of representing people.
   - New roles of the client council can be seen in monitoring and empowering direct feedback of clients to professionals and their systems.
   - Identify the main interest of patients: all patients have the right to be treated in a learning organization with as little as possible process-loss (the difference between what a group actually produces and what it might theoretically produce).

The study eventually led to the development of an almost costless feedback instrument that can be helpful to maximize the influence of clients within three circles of influence: 1. within the primary care process, 2. within the psychiatric clinics and 3. within the support services and board level of the organization.

To endorse the use of the feedback instrument, it was necessary to develop a structure and a method that together were able to work as a lever arch mechanism – a little power in combination with great movement will be converted into a small movement that transposes great power: 'Feedback in 1 minute'.

New model, new method

As a result, we made an effort to develop a direct form of co-determination. This is in line with contemporary research addressing this subject (Verwey-Jonker, 2015). In this study, co-determination is divided into formal (WMZC) and informal co-determination (no-WMCZ). Our research and instrument aim are based on two other dimensions: direct and indirect co-determination.

Basically, the need to increase knowledge about their disease is the reason why clients, as individuals, come to the institution. We concluded that this individual point of view must be the leading element in the work of the client council.

Method: *Feedback in 1 minute*

By creating the *Feedback in 1 minute*, we developed a short cyclic self-reflective and (self) evaluation instrument, to be used in the institution as a whole, in order to promote the learning capacities of clients and workers. So instead of there being a collective client council as an instrument of co-determination, we developed a one-person directed collective instrument which supports determination: from great movement and little power to little movement and great power. *Feedback in 1 minute* potentially applies to three levels in the organization: client-professional, supportive systems and clinics.

Feedback in 1 minute is an ultra-short questionnaire of four questions, two self-reflective and two feedback-oriented. The form and dynamics of this questionnaire were inspired by the slowly developing understanding that clients and workers should be strengthened to say on the spot what is needed to be said, in order to give full expression to the learning organization.

Short-cyclic instruments already exist in therapy settings. After we concluded that we wanted to create a mechanism for feedback on the spot, we started developing our ideas and after a while were drawn to the work of Anton Hafkenscheid (with whom we talked), Scott Miller and Barry Duncan (2010). After studying their type of short-cyclic feedback we concluded that our system in development stemmed from a different assumption. The *Feedback in 1 minute* we developed emphasizes the 'hard working client', who is active and takes his/her role in treatment. *Feedback in 1 minute* is not a fixed questionnaire, it varies. It is flexible and supports the phases in treatment. It supports making space to say the things that have to be said. The initiative to use the *Feedback in 1 minute* lies with the client. It is designed by clients for clients as a means to increase co-determination in three levels of the organization.

Feedback in 1 minute is shaped in the form of a folding card, it has no other use than to create awareness, reflection in actual context and make feedback possible. The person completing the feedback indicates their opinion about the propositions by marking on the dotted line, some 10 minutes before the end of the session/meeting. After doing this, the marks are discussed.

Primary process version

Feedback in 1 minute (primary process) is to be used during the primary process. Both client and professional have their own mirrored standard questionnaire. Used on the client's initiative, the professional version is on the back of the client's version.

The four questions relate to these dimensions:

1 Initiative, ownership/ be in charge of the subjects that need to be talked about.
2. Give/ask all information, needed to get/give right treatment.
3. Communication about the relationship of the client and staff member.
4. Opinion about effects of the used technique on recovery.

Clinic version

This is to be used during gatherings and meetings in clinics. Their questionnaire is partly standard, with one variable question to fill in about the ways the experience of the clients will be taken into account, to make 'nothing about us, without us' a reality.
The dimensions are:

1. Initiative, ownership, be in charge of the subjects that need to be talked about
2, How is client feedback obtained about subjects?
3. Communication about the relationship between clients and staff.
4. Opinion about effects and results of the meeting.

1. In this meeting I have raised all the subjects I intended to address.
No..Yes
2. Do we need to obtain direct client-feedback about the subjects we discussed in this meeting?
No..Yes
3. Did we communicate about the quality of our feedback and our relationships in this meeting?
No..Yes
4. This meeting has added value for the elements of the key focus of this organisation?
No..Yes
What will I do different next time?..

System and supporting services version.

The version for system/supporting services is used during gatherings, client council meetings, board meetings and staff meetings.
The dimensions are:

1. Initiative, ownership, be in charge of the subjects that need to be talked about.
2. How is value added for the clients of the organization?
3. Communication about the relationship between clients and staff
4. Opinion about effects and results of the meeting.

1. In this meeting I have raised all subjects I intended to address
No..Yes
2. This meeting has added value for the clients of the organization
No..Yes
3. Did we communicate about the quality of our feedback and our relationships in this meeting?
No..Yes
4. Does this meeting have added value for the elements of the key focus of this organisation?
No..Yes
What will I do different next time?..

To empower and structure the *Feedback in 1 minute* method we constructed a new structure which eventually can replace the client council model.

Model: task teams

The new model does not have the client council as the starting point of co-determination. The new starting point is the three rights of the WMCZ. Three autonomic task teams have been formed, they work as project groups and have their own budgets. The first team is the clinic-task team. These people are taking care of all subjects regarding the 'strengthened' WMCZ advice-questions. This team is responsible for arranging the feedback of clients of the clinics at the most direct level, they monitor the use of the new method *Feedback in 1 minute*-clinic.

The second task team is the system-task team. They are responsible for all ordinary WMCZ advice questions by the people working in supporting systems, CEO and management, and for all other rights and duties according to the WMCZ. Their responsibility is humanizing the systems within the organization. They do this by taking seats in committees, regarding quality, safety, and health issues and all other forms of policy making. The key issue will be: How do clients benefit from these meetings? This team monitors the *Feedback in 1 minute*-system.

The third task team is the initiative-task team. This task team is responsible for initiatives and advice that are not asked for. This task team is responsible for innovation in the field of the primary process; specifically being active in having a say in all possible situations within the health organization. This team monitors the *Feedback in 1 minute* (primary process).

Conclusion

In June 2020 the Dutch government published a specific guideline to support the new approach of the 2018 WMCZ. Article 2 of this new law decided that clients who need to reside in Mental Health facilities must have a direct say in their situation. Our *Feedback in 1 minute* instrument is recommended in this guideline as a useful vehicle in creating a genuine and effective culture of continue contact.

References

Benjamin, L. (1996) *Interpersonal Diagnosis and Treatment of Personality Disorders*. New York: The Guildford Press

Commissie van der Burg, (1977) *Rapport Van De Commissie Van Advies Inzake Het Democratisch En Doelmatig Functioneren Van Gesubsidieerde Instellingen (Report of the Advisory Committee on the Effective Functioning of Subsidized Institutions)*. The Hague: Staatsuitgeverij

Dijk, O, van der (2015) Motie nr.32012. 28. *Borgen van de medezeggenschap van patiënten en cliënten/ governance in de zorgsector (Motion for members: Governance in the healthcare sector)*

Guba, E. and Lincoln, Y. (1989) *Fourth Generation Evaluation*. Newbury Park, CA: Sage

Hafkenscheid, A., Duncan. B.L. and Miller, S.D. (2010) The outcome and session rating scales: A cross-cultural examination of the psychometric properties of the Dutch translation. *Journal Of Brief Therapy*, 7, 1&2

Heuts, P. (2015) Landelijke Organisatie Clienten (LOC)-raden in Tweede Kamer (Minutes of meeting with clientcouncils in Second chambre of Dutch Parliament)(29 mei 2015) *Zorg*

& Zeggenschap, uitgave 32, juni 2015, [Accessed 18 November 2016 at http://pienheuts.nl/wp-content/uploads/2015/07/ZZS-02-2015.pdf)

LCvV, landelijke Commissie van Vertrouwenslieden, [Accessed 18 November 2016 at http://vertrouwenslieden.actiz.ccilivits.nl/homepage]

Mein, A.G. and Oudenampsen, D. (2015) *Medezeggenschap op maat-Onderzoek naar de wijze waarop vorm en inhoud wordt gegeven aan medezeggenschap van cliënten in de zorg* (Co-determination with adequate impact-.Researching the ways of performing content with regard to clients in health care), Utrecht: Verwey-Jonker Instituut, [Accessed 18 November 2016 at http://www.verwey-jonker.nl/publicaties/2015/medezeggenschap-op-maat]

Research-team GGZ inGeest, (2017) Rapport Clientenraadsels (Report Clientenraadsels). Accessed 10 september 2022 at https//ncz/rapport-clientenraadsels.

Rijksoverheid, 2020 Inspraak in de WMCZ 2018, een handreiking voor zorgorganisaties en clientenraden (Clientparticipation in the WMCZ 2018, a guideline for healthorganizations and clientcouncils). rijksoverheid.nl

Thomson South-Western Wagner and Hollenbeck (n.d.) *Group Dynamics And Team Effectiveness*. [Accessed 11 July 2016 at http://slideplayer.com/slide/7832177/]

Trappenburg, M. (2004) *Lezing (lecture) Mentrum, Geestelijke gezondheidszorg (mental health). 28 October 2004*, [Accessed 18 November 2016 at http://margotrappenburg.nl/wp-content/uploads/2014/11/Lezing-voor-Mentrum.pdf]

Voet, G. van der (2005) *De kwaliteit van de WMCZ als medezeggenschapswet (The quality of the WMCZ as co-determination law)*. Erasmus School of Law (ESL). [Accessed 18 November 2016 at http://repub.eur.nl/pub/6920/]

Wetenschappelijke Raad Voor Het Regeringsbeleid (WRR) (2014) *Van tweeluik naar driehoeken, versterking van interne checks and balances bij semi-publieke organisaties (From dyptich to triangle. Strengthening internal checks and balances in semi-public organisations)*. Amsterdam: Amsterdam University Press, [Accessed 18 November 2016 at http://www.wrr.nl/fileadmin/nl/publicaties/PDF-rapporten/Van_tweeluik_naar_driehoek.pdf]

Wet Medezeggenschap Cliënten Zorginstellingen (WMCZ) (1996) *Medezeggenschap cliënten in de Zorg (Co –determination of clients in general health care)*. [Accessed 18 November 2016 at www.rijksoverheid.nl/onderwerpen/patientenrecht-en-clientenrecht/inhoud/medezeggenschap-clienten-in-de-zorg)

Wet Medezeggenschap Clienten Zorginstellingen (WMCZ 2018) Accessed 10 september 2022 at https//wetten.overheid.nl BWBROOO7920

Chapter 10
Educational vision quests of Canadian First Nations Youth:
A photovoice exploration

Debbie Laliberte Rudman, Chantelle Richmond, Treena Orchard and Anthony Isaac

This chapter shares results from a Canadian-based Photovoice project that examined issues related to inclusion of First Nations youth in post-secondary education (PSE). The project title, 'Educational Vision Quests,' evolved over time through the involvement of a First Nations Masters graduate student, Anthony Isaac. Based on his cultural understanding of a vision quest as 'a traditional Indigenous practice that provides a means to find one's gifts and obtain guidance on how to live a good life' (p.1), Isaac (2012) framed this project as a 'contemporary form of exploring the visions of First Nations youth in a culturally respectful manner' (p.1) that aimed to 'raise awareness of the facilitators and barriers encountered by Indigenous youth in the London, Ontario and surrounding area as they attempt to move forward in enacting PSE [post-secondary education]' (p.3).

Within this chapter, we describe the necessity of engaging in a strengths-based participatory process when addressing occupational injustices faced by Indigenous people, and outline the participatory process used in the Photovoice project. Drawing from the experiences of seven First Nations youth transitioning into or within post-secondary education, we outline how socio-political processes present challenges to progression and completion, as well as facilitators and supports. We discuss implications for building supports for First Nations students, as well as institutional changes required to optimize meaningful occupational engagement and expand occupational possibilities.

The necessity of a participatory approach

Globally, Indigenous people and communities have been and continue to be subjected to colonial practices aimed at assimilation, marginalization, degradation, erasure, and socio-political exclusion (Mowbray, 2007). In the face of such practices, Indigenous peoples and communities have often enacted resistance and demonstrated resilience; however, inequities related to income, health, housing, employment, access to social power, and many other socio-political determinants of social inclusion and health persist (Czyzewski, 2011; United Nations, 2009).

Within Canada, the Aboriginal population experiences many inter-related health and occupational inequities which are connected with colonial practices, experiences of inter-generational trauma, discrimination, and limited access to basic resources, among other factors (Frolich et al, 2006). For example, results from a 2011 survey indicate that Aboriginal Canadians have an unemployment rate more than twice that of the total Canadian population, and 9.8% completed university education compared to 26.5% of non-Aboriginal Canadians (Aboriginal Affairs and Northern Development Canada, 2015; Statistics Canada, 2014). It has been suggested that addressing such inequities is key to overcoming poverty, enhancing social capital, and advancing capacity for self-government and economic self-reliance (Reading & Wien, 2009).

As a means of addressing these inequities, the last decade has witnessed the development and uptake of a hopeful new research paradigm wherein Indigenous peoples themselves are taking control of research on their pressing concerns. Introduced by Maori scholar Linda Smith (1999), decolonizing methodologies are an approach to doing research that builds capacity for Indigenous self-determination and employs research as a way of Indigenous peoples re-gaining access to forms of power, tied to the capability to make decisions central to their lives and access resources required to enact control over their lives and destinies. As well, research historically has often failed to incorporate Indigenous worldviews, has often not been done in ways that have benefitted Aboriginal peoples and communities, and has been implicated in colonial practices (Mombray, 2007). Given this history and the recognition that research, particularly when coupled with action, can be a powerful tool to enact change by and with Indigenous communities, guidelines for conducting collaborative, respectful, mutually beneficial and ethical research premised on 'good relations' have been developed (Castellano & Reading, 2010). In the Canadian context, the First Nations Information Governance Committee produced an influential document, titled 'OCAP: Ownership, Control, Access and Possession' (First Nations Centre, 2007) that provides guidance for communities and researchers to 'make decisions regarding what research will be done, for what purpose information or data will be used, where the information will be physically stored and who will have access' (p.1).

The necessity of enacting a participatory approach is heightened when addressing issues of social inclusion. Given long-standing efforts of Indigenous peoples to resist assimilation and maintain Indigenous ways of knowing and doing, efforts aimed at combating social exclusion must avoid assuming inclusion into the 'mainstream' as a desired endpoint. Thus, 'efforts to counter 'social exclusion' must be informed by a close understanding of Indigenous peoples' particular circumstances and perspectives' (Mombray, 2007, p.30). There must be a constant awareness of how historical assimilationist practices were often justified with the stated intent of inclusion and, in turn, a commitment to de-constructing, re-configuring and diversifying what have been taken-for-granted as 'mainstream' ways of doing.

Getting started

The Educational Vision Quests project occurred in London, Ontario, Canada. London has a population of about 400,000 residents, and is a regional centre for health care and post-secondary education (PSE). Within Canada, the Aboriginal population is comprised of three groups, the First Nations, the Inuit and the Métis; each of which occupy distinctive territories, speak different languages, and follow unique cultural practices. First Nations peoples comprise the largest Indigenous peoples in Canada and in London there are about 6,000 First Nations people living in the city, and some 34,000 living on 'reserve' communities and rural areas within commuting distance (Assembly of First Nations, n.d.; Statistics Canada, 2006). Reserve communities were a colonial practice that began in the mid-1800s that involved placing First Nations peoples into bounded pieces of land, and having them give up their land rights through imbalanced treaty negotiations. Historically, the government set limitations on travel outside of these communities and the occupations First Nations people could do within such communities, including cultural practices related to hunting, dancing and spirituality. While such limitations no longer exist, reserve communities do, with First Nations people living both on and off reserve. Moreover, pervasive problems persist in terms of access to a variety of essential resources, ranging from clean water to educational opportunities, within many reserve communities (Browne et al, 2005; Frolich et al., 2006).

Ideally, enacting a participatory approach begins with defining the focus of a project. Practically, enacting a participatory approach from the initiation of a project can be challenging, particularly when a group does not have a pre-existing history of working together (Cargo & Mercer, 2008). In this project, in order to secure resources to support in-depth discussions with members of local First Nations communities and organizations, several university-based investigators applied for project development funding from a government source interested in 'human capital' development. As such, the initiation of the project was bounded within the notion of 'human capital' research as defined by this funding body to include 'research and innovation projects that identify better ways to help people prepare for, return to or keep employment and become productive participants in the labour force' (http://www.tcu.gov.on.ca/eng/eopg/programs/ohcrif.html). At the same time, part of the rationale for applying to this funding body was that various Indigenous organizations and scholars in the Canadian context have identified inequities in education and labour market opportunities as key issues needing to be addressed in order to build community capacity for self-governance and address long-standing social and health inequities (Loppie Reading & Wein, 2009; Richmond & Ross, 2009). Working within this broad focus, we subsequently attempted to remain open to issues voiced by representatives of local Indigenous communities and organizations and to be critically mindful of the need for educational and work institutions to shift away from being means of assimilation towards being means to foster capacity building and self-determination (Stonechild, 2006).

Once funding was obtained, we hosted two, open discussion meetings with various local First Nations communities, local First Nations organizations whose mandate included issues relevant to education and labour force involvement, and First Nations undergraduate and graduate students. The primary purposes of these meetings were to: a) explore the possibility of working together on a project, b) discuss local issues related to the 'human capital' development of First Nations peoples, and c) delineate a focus for a collaborative project. As the meetings occurred, a fourth purpose, related to defining guiding principles, emerged. This purpose evolved as the group discussed the centrality of maintaining 'good relations', and also because many First

Nations' representatives expressed that it was unlikely they could sustain involvement over the project time frame of a year to two years. These representatives expressed that committing to a project over such a time frame was challenging, given that the funding basis for their key service activities and human resources were unstable and required them to prioritize on-going efforts to ensure sustainability. Thus, given the value they attributed to the project, they desired to have input into the principles that would guide it as we moved forward.

During the first meeting, the group agreed that a participatory project was feasible, and that a focus on inequities in education for First Nations youth, particularly PSE, could provide promising, relevant information. Within the second meeting, the group explored various types of methodologies, and reached agreement on visual methods. Photography was identified as a particularly useful approach to engage Indigenous youth and provide an opportunity for skill development, as well as creative expression of their PSE experiences. The dialogue led to the generation of five guiding project principles: a) create space for youths' perspectives; b) integrate Indigenous ways of knowing and doing; c) learn and do collaboratively; d) examine social conditions that shape possibilities for PSE; and e) use the results to promote promising practices. At the end of these meetings, our research team consisted of: representatives from the Southwestern Ontario Aboriginal Health Access Centre (SOAHAC), N'Amerind Friendship Centre, and Indigenous Services at Western; a First Nations graduate student; an interdisciplinary team of researchers from the University of Western Ontario, including a First Nations scholar; and an Indigenous educational advocate from a nearby university. Although the diversity of our research team would have been enhanced via the participation of members representing local First Nations Reserve communities, the organizations involved had pre-existing partnerships with these communities in various ways and thus were able to provide knowledge about these communities.

Placing the 'local issue' and refining our research aims

To move forward in addressing the issue of inequities in PSE, we first placed this locally identified issue within the broader Canadian context. The knowledge gained was used to craft a research proposal and obtain funding. A review of various types of literature, including that produced by Indigenous organizations and published peer-reviewed articles, made the extent of the locally identified problem clear: educational disparities between Indigenous and non-Indigenous Canadians have been identified as a significant social and health issue (Canadian Council on Learning, 2006). As well, this contemporary problem is rooted in history and its continuing effects. In particular, education was a key occupational means of assimilation. Beginning in mid-1800s and continuing in some places until the mid-1990s, a residential school system was enacted based on the assumption that the best way for First Nations children to succeed would be to ban them from learning traditional ways of knowing and doing and focus education on Canadian customs, Christianity and English or French (Smith et al, 2005). At the same time, numerous Indigenous scholars and organizations have proposed that if education can be shifted from a tool of assimilation to one for capacity building, it is a key way forward in enhancing the well-being and self-determination of First Nations peoples (Canadian Council on Learning, 2006; Stonechild, 2006).

Applying an occupational perspective, these long-standing educational inequities were framed as a situation of occupational injustice (Wilcock & Townsend, 2000), in that social, economic, political, historical and other conditions have created situations in which many Indigenous peoples cannot enact the right to education, particularly within environments which were not based on principles of assimilation.

Drawing upon what we had learned through exploratory meetings, further dialogue amongst the research team members, and the literature, we refined our research aims to include: a) increase understandings of the strengths, assets and needs of First Nations youth in relation to PSE experiences and visions of success, and b) increase awareness of supports and barriers (including the ways educational institutions can be assimilationist in their aims and practices) encountered by First Nations youth in London, Ontario and surrounding area as they attempt to move forward in PSE.

Designing our methodology and methods

Photovoice is a critically informed qualitative methodology that incorporates participant-generated photography to mutually create knowledge, facilitate dialogue and inform strategies for change (Wang & Burris, 1997). In a typical photovoice study, photos are taken and discussed within a group context (Asaba et al, 2015). To adhere to the guiding principle of incorporating Indigenous ways of knowing and doing, and also to optimize cultural safety and respect for the First Nations youth collaborators, we modified photovoice methodology. Specifically, modifications included, and were informed by, the involvement of three First Nations Elders who were present at all project events and provided on-going consultation from development of the ethics protocol to the photo exhibit. For example, similar to Castleden, H., Garvin, T., and Huu-ay-aht First Nations (2008), the Elders expressed concern that bringing individually-generated photos to a focus group discussion might be threatening to youth and advised that we provide an opportunity for youth to talk through photos on an individual basis prior to choosing what to bring forth to a group.

Our study was comprised of five main phases: recruitment, photovoice training, photo taking and individual interviews, focus group, and photo exhibit and community celebration. Informed by a strengths-based perspective, we recruited seven First Nations youth who were in the final stages of secondary school or transitioning into a PSE program. Recruitment was done primarily through hosting an information session at N'Amerind Friendship Centre. In the Photovoice training session, the study purpose was discussed, Elders shared traditional teachings, a photographer provided education, and the youth established collective guidelines for group interaction. The Elders drew parallels between traditional teachings related to valuing experiential knowledge, learning through doing and learning about one's place in the world to the aims and approaches being used in the Photovoice project. This was followed by the photo-taking phase, varying in length according to how the youth chose to participate, wherein youth took photos with a supplied camera that conveyed their visions of educational success and barriers and facilitators of their visions. Each youth then participated in an individual qualitative interview, and all the youth participated in a subsequent focus group for which each youth collaborator chose three photos. The focus group purpose was to engage the youth in a dialogue to collectively identify the broader conditions shaping PSE experiences and aspirations. The final stage was a photo exhibit at the Friendship Centre. Following the exhibit, the people invited, including the youth, their significant others, other research team members, local elders, other community organizations, and educational representatives from various institutions, shared in a community celebration, and discussed the photos and action strategies aimed at enhancing educational possibilities for First Nations youth.

As a methodology, Photovoice was designed to acknowledge and value the capacities of collaborators as agents, while simultaneously enhancing awareness of social conditions and processes that perpetuate oppression and marginalization (Asaba et al, 2015). For example, co-reflections and consulting with Elders led to the inclusion of a pipe ceremony and community celebration with the Photo exhibit, as a means to provide a space to honor youth and promote community dialogue. Although we worked to ensure on-going incorporation of participatory principles through the study process, for example, by ensuring youth made choices about their photos, we found it difficult to sustain a fully participatory approach in the analysis process given the time commitment required. Analysis was primarily carried out by the four authors of this chapter. It involved inductive coding of interview and focus group transcripts, as well as photos, and abductive coding informed by concepts drawn from occupational science, critical social theory, and Indigenous scholarship. For each youth, Anthony constructed a narrative of his or her articulated educational journey that integrated his or her words and photos; this was provided back to the youth. As well, dialogue that occurred in the community celebration and amongst the research team regarding photos and emerging findings further informed analysis.

Introducing our youth collaborators

The youth collaborators included 4 females and 3 males, aged 17 to 29 years of age, who self-identified as belonging to the Oneida, Chippewa, Delaware, Anishinabe, and Mohawk Nations1. They were at various points in their PSE journeys; some were finishing high school, some were in the first year of PSE, and some were re-attempting PSE following previous uncompleted attempts. They were enrolled in and applying for different types of PSE, and had a variety of life situations. Within this chapter, each youth is identified with a pseudonym.

Summarizing lessons learned

We frame the study 'findings' as lessons learned through the participatory process of engaging with the youth collaborators. Contrary to assumptions about First Nations youth as not motivated to participate in education that sometimes inform research and media, the youth in this study discussed education as both an individual and collective necessity and passion. PSE was described as something they had to do in order to survive, given the limited opportunities available to them within their current lives, and as providing opportunities to advance possibilities for themselves, their families, and their communities. Jasmine, who was in the final stages of completing her high school diploma after having dropped out when a teenager, explained how education provided a way to move forward:

> *'I was working for a little bit and then I realized like, what am I doing? Like I'm not even doing like anything, just at home. Still living with my parents, living off of minimum wage, so...I'm going back to school...now a days you can't do anything unless you're educated.'*

Spencer, who moved from his reserve community to attend a college in London, discussed how education was connected to both individual and community development. Reflecting on a picture of a sun rise, Spencer described education as 'coming out of the darkness' and as helping him see the 'light of the new day'. Spencer, like many of the youth collaborators, had a strong connection to his home community and framed education as providing a way to enhance one's capacities to contribute to community development,

> *'once I complete all [of my aspirations], then maybe I can get a job back in the community or in a different community where I can help their community out somehow.'*

Emma also framed education as essential for continued development of First Nations communities; reflecting on a picture of a building which had been a residential school, she stated,

> *'It was a bad time and we just have to overcome it and do better. They need native politicians, they need all these people in respective positions, but you need education to get there right?'*

Several youth described themselves as contributing to their communities by being a mentor; as stated by Alana, 'I'd hope that [youth] would look toward somebody who has done something with their life...Just if I do something, just for them to see there are [opportunities]'.

Second, the youth provided insight into particular social conditions, relations and practices that need to be addressed to enhance possibilities for education. Spencer, Emma, Alana and Bailey all discussed challenges associated with leaving their homes and communities, located on reserves, but also how they had faced limited opportunities within these communities. For example, reflecting on photos of the landscape of her community, Bailey stated,

> *'These are pictures of my favourite places in the world...where I am originally from. I miss it there a lot...I always contemplate moving back home...but I don't want to because there is nothing there for my own education.'*

As a second example of socially located challenges, the youth discussed broadly accepted negative perceptions of Indigenous people, and how racism influenced their educational pursuits. Lex, reflecting on a photo of his shadow, discussed facing racism and stereotypes as an everyday part of life for First Nations peoples, 'everyone else's preconceived notions of us [referring to Indigenous youth] will always follow us, like a shadow'. Bailey also discussed having to deal with negative stereotypes,

> *'there are certain things that everyone still has to overcome. Like even in education...those kind of stereotypes I remember hearing when I was little...when I was going to school.'*

As a final example, there has been a long-standing silence within educational and other institutions in Canada regarding colonial practices and their enduring effects. The youth expressed that not knowing this history sometimes led First Nations youth to internalize broader, negative stereotypes and believe that their possibilities for education were necessarily limited. They also discussed how they had to go outside of the mainstream educational system to learn about their history in ways that acknowledged the strengths of Indigenous peoples, with most of them learning this history through local Indigenous organizations or family members. Reflecting on a photo of the 'Mush Hole', a nickname for a local, former residential school, Emma stressed the need for Indigenous youth to know their history to move forward in positive ways,

> 'A majority of us are a product of a generation or two from this residential school. …. We want to show our youth where they come from because some of them are starting to be adults, go into school, and go to Universities, College, and all that stuff. Some of them do not know where they come from. They do not know their history and I think it is important to know your history.'

Third, a very strong thread tying the stories together was that the youth understood their abilities to negotiate challenges faced in their educational journeys to having foundational ties to culture, families and ancestral history. While previous research on factors predicting low educational attainment has often focused on negative characteristics of Indigenous families, the youth collaborators discussed family support, in combination with support drawn from culture and ancestral history, as key to providing them with a strong sense of who they were that enabled them to push forward. For example, reflecting on a photo of a tree which he had titled 'strong roots support growth', Lex emphasized how his roots as 'Native' were solidified by engaging in traditional fasting with his father.

> 'Luckily, I was able to fast and stuff with my dad at a young age so I could set the roots in like a tree and know exactly what I want to do and have a strong foundation. So that way I can grow upward a lot more easily and not have to be confused at what I wanted.'

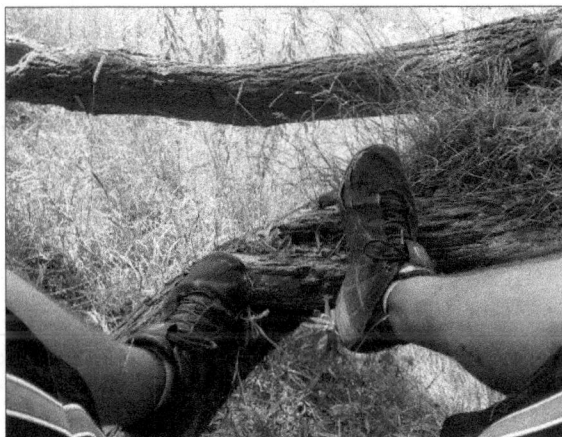

Fig 1. Strong roots

Similarly, Spencer, reflecting on a picture of his feet standing on tree roots, discussed his family, as well as his cultural knowledge, as foundational,

'if you know your heritage, if you know your culture, that's something you can learn. You can use that as your guide or you can use that to move forward in your life. When you do meet obstacles or something, then you have that background behind you to kinda fall back on, and then it can help you push forward'.

Several youth discussed the importance of encountering places, such as First Nations Centres in educational institutions, people, such as Elders and First Nations mentors who had completed education, and occupations, such as dancing, art and sports, that connected them to Indigenous ways of knowing and doing.

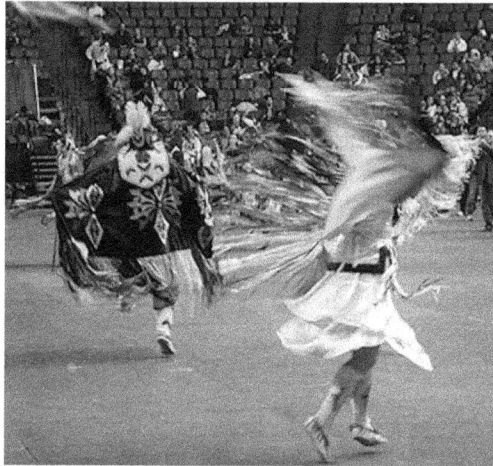

Fig 2. Balance through dancing

For example, Emma, reflecting on a picture of herself engaged in a traditional dance stated:

'This one [represents] healing because there's a story behind the jingle dresses...You need that stuff in school. Like, if sometimes you just had a tough week or a tough month or a tough semester and you have to deal with all this stuff while you're going to school...you just gotta find these things that help you cope with it. '

Spencer discussed how he had become more engaged in cultural occupations when he finished high school, and expressed that this made it 'not as difficult to succeed',

'I started learning with my own cousin, and that's what he did right out of high school. He was always learning like the culture...I started with singing and dancing, and then slowly made it into the ceremonies, and I'm starting to learning ceremonies and how they are conducted.'

Finally, a pervasive finding was that challenges to maintaining a strong sense of identity as an Indigenous person arose from being within an educational system, and broader society, that devalues, or ignores, Indigenous ways of knowing and doing.

Alana, reflecting on a picture of a tree in the Fall, discussed dealing with the possibility that education might try to assimilate First Nations youth, an awareness rooted in interactions with those who had been, or whose parents had been, in residential schools. Alana stated,

'Some people's views against education might be like…'they're going to try and conform me to be like the white people' and stuff like that. I don't think education is going change…I think that it's us that has to…live in the white world, but remember in our heart where we come from…or where we belong…. where our home is. Our home, our traditions, our culture… Like as long as [education] doesn't change who you are, then I think it's okay to learn the same thing as everybody else.'

The youth noted that committing to cultural ways of knowing and doing and maintaining an identity as Indigenous was a continuous tension, a tension shaped and perpetuated through their experiences within an educational system in which, as Lex said, they felt like they were 'living in the shadows'. The youth spoke of needing to negotiate a balance between Indigenous and Western ways of doing and knowing, and of feeling, in Spencer's words, that they were 'in between" and facing a 'dilemma between your today and then your traditional culture as well, because it always seems like you're fighting yourself whether to be this way or whether to be that way'.

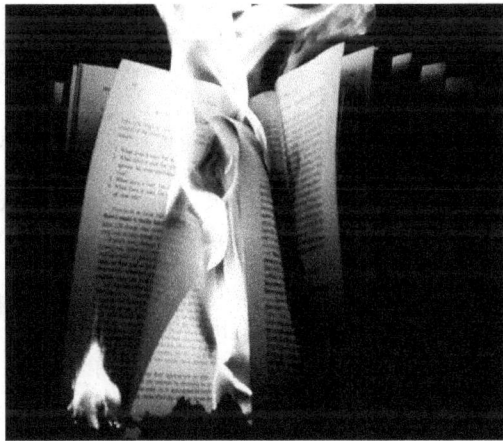

Fig 4. A classic affirmation

As another example, unlike other participants who took many photos, Mitchell, who had struggled in high school and resented being failed in courses, took just one photo of a burning book. Reflecting on his identity struggles, Mitchell stated,

'Well, my father's Oneida. And my mother's Chippewa. So…you know that just adds to the frustration. Like what I am? But I'm here [in London] too. And plus, the society we live in…

it's like identity. Am I supposed to believe, am I supposed to have this culture? Just thinking about it – like trying to give myself identity – gives me stress...You just try to live within this society, try to work with it – just do it.'

Implications and moving forward

Promoting social inclusion requires the dismantling of barriers to the equitable participation of all members of a society in diverse spheres of public life (Labonte, 2004), in concert with the implementation of structural and system level change that works against assimilationist agendas and ensures inclusivity and valuing of diversity (Truth and Reconciliation Commission of Canada, 2015). Within this study, participants identified several factors that challenged PSE involvement. These challenges included various forms of racism, as well as exclusionary institutional practices in educational settings that marginalized Indigenous knowledge and practices. Our youth collaborators shared how various factors created a sense of being 'in between' cultures, which challenged the ways they negotiate their identities, as well as how such factors operated in ways that marginalized them within and from educational institutions. At the same time, the youth emphasized how foundational supports, connected to family, history and culture, and engagement in occupations that connected them with their culture, enabled them to pursue educational pursuits that promoted their growth and that of their communities.

The findings highlight the vital need for PSE educators and administrators to acknowledge the negative history of assimilationist educational policies in Canada, and to critically reflect on how these policies have shaped their programs and educational practices. This is required to make education more affirming of Indigenous identity; for example, through integrating and valuing Indigenous ways of knowing and doing with programs, services, and curricula. As well, it is important to acknowledge the presence of racism, and revise policies and programs to enhance cultural inclusivity and continuously work against everyday and systemic racism. Working with Indigenous communities and organizations, post-secondary institutions need to foster and support spaces on campuses that provide Indigenous youth with places to engage in valued ways of doing and being, and to interact with each other and Elders to share experiences of, and negotiate, the experience of being 'in between'. As well, as articulated in the recommendations put forth by the recently released report of the Truth and Reconciliation Commission in Canada (2015), post-secondary institutions, in partnership with Indigenous students, communities and organizations, need to ensure that all students are exposed to educational opportunities that enhance awareness of the historical and on-going impact of colonial practices in the Canadian context and promote inter-cultural dialogue and mutual respect.

In many ways our youth collaborators affirmed various directions forwarded by several Indigenous organizations in Canada, as well by our community partners, as key ways forward in supporting First Nations youth (Canadian Council on Learning, 2008). In addition, our study showed how such directions can sustain youths' efforts to move ahead in educational vision quests. These directions include: providing opportunities for First Nations youth to engage in Indigenous ways of doing as a means to learn about Indigenous culture and build a strong sense of identity; providing places within PSE environments that foster a sense of belonging in the broader Indigenous community, enabling a sense of 'home' and family; and providing opportunities to connect with, and become, mentors among Indigenous youth. Such initiatives need to occur in concert with the broader institutional systems noted above, so that Indigenous youth are not 'othered' via taking up opportunities to affirm and enact Indigenous ways of knowing and doing.

Arising out of the project, various team members have become involved in activities aimed at raising awareness of how educational and related inequities are socially perpetuated, and facilitating discussion regarding how to support educational possibilities for First Nations youth and how to raise the knowledge and awareness of all students regarding the historical and contemporary socio-political determinants of Indigenous health and well-being. For example, members contributed to a task force in the Faculty of Health Sciences at Western University, which was co-led by a community representative from N'Amerind Friendship Centre. Activities of the task force included evaluating undergraduate students' current knowledge and attitudes related to Indigenous history, culture and health, and forwarding recommendations for the inclusion of Indigenous knowledge and history with curricula as well as the creation of spaces for Indigenous faculty and students within various educational programs. In the School of Occupational Therapy, for example, educational sessions on the history of Indigenous peoples within Canada were provided by a First Nations educational consultant to all of the occupational therapy students, and two spots in the program were set aside for Indigenous students. In addition, several members of the research team, including representatives from SOAHAC, collaborated on a project that provided opportunities for First Nations youth, aged 10 to 12, to engage in Indigenous ways of doing and learn Indigenous knowledge. This project , the *Bimaadiziwin ('good life') Learning Experience*, was led by First Nations youth counsellors; incorporated various types of occupations, such as traditional crafts, a medicine walk and interactions with elders; and also involved an MSc student in Occupational Science, Klya English, completing an arts-based inquiry to enhance understandings of childrens' perceptions of health (English, 2014). Engagement in these various participatory projects has further solidified the team's on-going collaboration within an on-going research-action cycle to address issues that Indigenous peoples and communities experience as key to health and well-being.

In relation to occupation-based social inclusion, this project provides an example of how critical qualitative methodologies can be taken up to unpack how occupational injustices are shaped, negotiated and enacted. In turn, such enhanced understanding can facilitate the capacity of occupational therapists and scientists, working in collaboration with communities and across disciplines, to critique, raise awareness of and change socio-political conditions that form, perpetuate and justify occupational injustices. Although raising awareness is only one type of social action, it is foundational to other forms given the need to 'awaken the reader's sense of obligation to transform social injustice rather than simply watch it unfold' (Blustein et al, 2012, p.349). We end this chapter with a reflective quote from Spencer, who encapsulated the importance of awareness raising:

'Me and Anthony had to sit down for like four hours like during lunch just talking about it [his photos and education]. But it made me feel good after talking, and explaining about the pictures. Sometimes I was just taking pictures, and I just looked back and then, and I was like, yeah, that means something to me, to my success, to my education. Hopefully it means something to somebody else, all these pictures that we're all doing. Hopefully people can get an understanding of how it is to be Aboriginal, and trying to go to school.'

Note

1. 'First Nations' people are one of three 'Aboriginal' groups recognized in the Canadian constitution. First Nations people encompass almost 1 million people who belong to over 50 different linguistic and cultural groups, with these groups varying by geographic region. (https://www.rcaanc-cirnac.gc.ca/eng/1100100013785/1529102490303). Within the province of Ontario, there are approximately 13 distinct First Nations groups (Spotton, 2006).

Acknowledgements

This project, as a participatory endeavor, had many contributors. We wish to acknowledge the work of Anthony Isaac, who played a vital role in designing and enacting this study, and who has contributed to this manuscript based on his on continuing Vision Quest. We also acknowledge the commitment to the project of the seven youth collaborators and the Elders who provided on-going support, and the directors and various staff members of the Southwest Ontario Aboriginal Health Access Centre, N'Amerind Friendship Centre and Indigenous Services at Western. We acknowledge funding support from the Ontario Ministry of Training, Colleges and Universities, and the Social Sciences and Research Council of Canada. Additional co-investigators on these grants include Suzanne Huot, Lisa Klinger, Lilian Magalhaes, Angela Mandich, Lynn Shaw, Darren Thomas, and Jerry White. Formal ethics approval was obtained from the University of Western Ontario, and on-going dialogue about how to conduct the study in ways that maintained good relations occurred amongst the research team and participating Elders.

References

Asaba, E., Laliberte Rudman, D., Mondaca, M. and Park, M. (2015) Visual methodologies – Photovoice in focus. in S. Nayar and M. Stanley (Eds.) *Qualitative Research Methodologies for Occupational Science And Occupational Therapy*. New York, NY: Routledge (pp.155-173)

Aboriginal Affairs and Northern Development Canada (2015) *Fact Sheet - 2011 National Household Survey Aboriginal Demographics, Educational Attainment and Labour Market Outcomes*. [Accessed 22 April 2022 at https://www.sac-isc.gc.ca/eng/1376329205785/1604610645621]

Assembly of Nations (n.d.) *Fact Sheet: First Nations Population* [Accessed 28 April 2015 at http://www.afn.ca/article.asp?id=2918]

Blustein, D.L., Medvide, M.B. and Wan, C.M. (2012) A critical perspective of contemporary unemployment policies and practices. *Journal of Career Development*, 39, 4, 341-356

Browne, A.J., Syme, V.L. and Varcoe, C. (2005) The relevance of postcolonial theoretical perspectives to research in Aboriginal health. *Canadian Journal on Nursing Research*, 37, 4, 16-37

Canadian Council on Learning (2008) *Post-Secondary Education: In support of First Nations and Inuit students.* Calgary, Alberta

Castleden, H., Garvin, T., and Huu-ay-aht First Nation (2008) Modifying photovoice for community-based participatory Indigenous research. *Social Science & Medicine*, 66, 6, 1393-1405

Castellano, M.B. and Reading, J. (2010) Policy writing as dialogue: Drafting an Aboriginal chapter for Canada's Tri-Council statement: Ethical conduct for research involving humans. *The International Indigenous Policy Journal*, 1, 2, Article 1 [Accessed 3 April 2015 at http://ir.lib.uwo.ca/iipj/vol1/iss2/1.]

Cargo, M. and Mercer, S.L. (2008) The value and challenges of participatory research: Strengthening its practice. *Annual Review of Public Health*, 29, 325-350

Czyzekski, K. (2011) Colonialism as a broader social determinant of health. *The International Indigenous Policy Journal*, 2,1, Article 5 [Accessed 3 April 2015 at http://ir.lib.uwo.ca/iipj/vol2/issue1/5]

English, K. (2014) *Through the eyes of children: First Nations children's perceptions of health.* Unpublished Masters thesis, University of Western Ontario, London, Ontario, Canada

First Nations Centre (2007). *OCAP: Ownership, Control, Access and Possession.* Sanctioned by the First Nations Information Governance Committee, Assembly of First Nations. Ottawa: National Aboriginal Health Organization

Frolich, K.L., Ross, N. and Richmond, C. (2006) Health disparities in Canada today: some evidence and a theoretical framework. *Health Policy*, 79, 132-143

Isaac, A. (2012) *Educational vision quests: Using Photovoice to explore the perspectives of First Nations Youth during their transition to post-secondary education.* Unpublished Masters thesis, University of Western Ontario, London, Ontario, Canada

Labonte, R. (2004) Social inclusion/exclusion: Dancing the dialectic. *Health Promotion International*, 19, 1, 115-121

Loppie Reading, C. & Wien, F. (2009). *Health inequalities and the social determinants of Aboriginal Peoples' Health.* Ottawa, Ontario: National Collaborating Centre on Aboriginal health

Mowbray, M. (2007) *Report on the International Symposium on the Social Determinants of Indigenous Health for the Commission on Social Determinants of Health – Social determinants and Indigenous health: The international experience and policy implications.* Sydney, Australia: Commission on Social Determinants of Health. [Accessed 21 April 2022 at https://humanrights.gov.au/about/news/speeches/social-determinants-and-health-indigenous-peoples-australia-human-rights-based

Reading, C.L. and Wein, F. (2009) *Health inequities and social determinants of Aboriginal people's health.* Prince George, British Columbia: National Collaborating Centre for Aboriginal Health. [Accessed 3 June 2011 at http://www.nccah-ccnsa.ca/docs/social%20determinates/NCCAH-Loppie-Wien_Report.pdf]

Richmond, C.A.M. and Ross, N.A. (2009) The determinants of First Nation and Inuit health: A critical population health approach. *Health Place*, 15, 2, 403-411

Smith, D., Varcoe, C., and Edwards, N. (2005) Turning around the intergenerational impact of residential schools on Aboriginal people: Implications for health policy and practice. *Canadian Journal of Nursing Research*, 37, 4, 38-60

Smith, L. T. (1999) *Decolonizing methodologies: Research and indigenous peoples.* London, UK: Zed Books

Spotton, N. (2006). *A profile of Aboriginal Peoples in Ontario.* Ontario: Ipperwash Inquiry.

Statistics Canada (2006). *2006 Aboriginal Population Profiles for Selected Cities and Communities* (London) [Accessed 3 June 2010 at http://www.statcan.gc.ca/bsolc/olc-cel/olc-cel?catno=89-638-X&lang=eng&chropg=1]

Statistics Canada (2014) *The educational attainment of Aboriginal peoples in Canada.* [Accessed 15 April 2015 at http://www12.statcan.gc.ca/nhs-enm/2011/as-sa/99-012-x/99-012-x2011003_3-eng.pdf]

Stonechild, B. (2006) *The new buffalo: The struggle for Aboriginal post-secondary education in Canada.* Winnipeg, Manitoba: University of Manitoba Press

Truth and Reconciliation Commission of Canada (2015) *Honouring the truth, reconciling for the future: Summary of the final report of the Truth and Reconciliation Commission of Canada.* Winnipeg, Manitoba: Truth and Reconciliation Commission of Canada

United Nations, Department of Economics and Social Affairs (2009) *State of the World's Indigenous peoples. New York: United Nations.* [Accessed 5 April 2010 at http://www.un.org/esa/socdev/ unpfii/ documents/SOWIP_web.pdf]

Wang, C. and Burris, M.A. (1997) Photovoice: Concept, methodology, and use for participatory needs assessment. *Health Education Behaviour*, 24, 3, 369-387

Wilcock, A.A. and Townsend, E.A. (2010) Occupational justice. *Journal of Occupational Science*, 7,2, 84-86

Chapter 11
'Occupy research': Research as socially inclusive occupation

Natasha Layton, Ricky Buchanan, Erin Wilson

Introduction: Who are we anyway?

There are several ways we can introduce ourselves to you as chapter authors. Ricky is disabled; Natasha is an occupational therapist and Erin her PhD supervisor [1]. This is not the whole story, but we have each selected labels to represent the identity we speak from in this instance. Using labels in this way may have already positioned us in certain ways in your eyes as the reader. In fact, the concept of disabled as 'other' is not one we are comfortable with, as we all identify as people subject to some human variation or other, on the wide spectrum of human diversity. It is also accurate to describe Ricky as an active blogger, web designer and advocate who has mentored Natasha and Erin in her lived experience of chronic illness, which is so severe that Ricky largely lives and works from her bed. We became collaborators and then colleagues through our various roles in *The Equipping Inclusion Studies* (Layton et al, 2010), a set of Australian studies into the costs and outcomes of assistive technologies and related supports.

This chapter is about the research experience from the perspectives of researcher and researched person, framed in the context of emancipatory and participatory research literature. We demonstrate that:

- Doing research involves multiple occupations
- Doing research can be empowering, health promoting and an action of social inclusion
- Doing research should be within reach of those who are the subjects of research.
- We argue that inclusion in research, in its widest sense, is a social justice issue. To understand the importance of social inclusion it is helpful to consider what social exclusion looks like

'An individual is socially excluded if (a) he or she is geographically resident in a society and (b) he or she does not participate in the normal activities of citizens in that society' (Burchardt, Le Grand & Piachaud, 1999, p. 230).

Social inclusion is about participation in socially valued and valuable occupational roles, research being one of these. Disabled people have infrequently participated in the array of key research activities which make up being a researcher and doing research. If social inclusion results from participation in occupations, and if the occupation of research is one from which disabled people have been excluded, then the act of *occupying* research is an act of social justice. We propose that occupying research is an aspect of social inclusion as it values and affirms the research roles of disabled people, and is a mechanism by which they produce knowledge. Based on this idea we provide some practical suggestions regarding how to occupy research.

The research project upon which we base our discussion was co-constructed by people living with disability, university-based researchers, assistive technology practitioners and advocates. This co-production approach came about when a community alliance of stakeholders (The Aids and Equipment Action Alliance)[2] gained philanthropic funding for a research project. Co-production brought with it a range of interesting issues. One was the need to separate systemic advocacy aims from data collection and analysis. Another was the complexity of gaining ethical approval when participants wished to own their data.

The co-production approach also enabled people to collaborate and learn from each other. For some of our 100 participants, their engagement with the research process went well beyond traditional respondent role, and this was an unexpected but welcome outcome. In this research project, participation in research for people with disability became an occasion of occupation-based social inclusion. Occupation, here, means participating in, producing and disseminating research. Occupying research in this way meant people were included in a community of researchers as authors and advocates with something to say. For some participants, this was a profound experience of social inclusion in an important and serious endeavour, as will be described. This chapter explores perspectives on the occupation of research from the viewpoint of research subject/agent (Ricky) and appointed researcher (Natasha and Erin).

Research as occupation

Participation in research by research subjects is not often framed as occupation. We argue here that this framing helps us understand participation in research, and enhances the valuing of individuals who choose to spend their time in this way.

The term occupation refers to all purposeful human activity (Wilcock, 1998). Occupation critically influences health and well-being (Law et al, 1998), and social inclusion is a core outcome of valued occupations (World Bank, 2013). Occupation is critical to our identity (Unruh, 2004) and to self-actualisation, whether it is an immediate experience of a single occupation, or dynamic and lifelong engagements with a range of occupations (Persson et al, 2001). The occupational deprivation and social inclusion literature illustrates that all humans need environments which provide opportunity to engage in occupations (Whiteford, 2011). Limited occupational roles and opportunities lead to occupational deprivation: an experience prevalent among people with disability (Whiteford, 2011). The historic and pervasive devaluing of the lives and roles of people living with disability means that, as well as the *opportunity* to engage, disabled people also require affirmation of the *value* of their occupational engagement (Rebeiro, 2001).

These ideas have important implications for thinking about research participation for people who are framed as subjects of research, including people with disability. Being a subject within a research project is very different from being an agent or active director of research. Participation in the occupation of research, can provide meaning, identity and, potentially, health and wellbeing outcomes. As Trentham and Cockburn (2005) argue,

> 'when people ask questions, propose solutions, implement change and disseminate new knowledge they are participating in an occupational form that helps to develop the skills and knowledge necessary to take greater control over their own lives; in doing so, they promote their own health as well as the health of other community members.' (Trentham & Cockburn, 2005, p.446)

The way we design research should be critically examined to show the extent to which it denies opportunities for occupational engagement. The research occupations or roles we make available to participants should also be examined for the quality and value of engagement they offer. For example, filling in a survey counts as a research engagement, but it is likely to offer a very different experience of occupational fulfilment compared with consulting on the relevance of an overarching research question to one's life (Jones, Ben-David, & Hole, 2020).

Research roles

Generally speaking, research is performed by researchers, that is, professional people with research credentials who are associated with various research institutions. Most research literature, presents a mainstreamed and ordered system in which researcher / researched roles are clearly delineated, and the researcher has more power. The idea of participation in research by the *researched* or research subjects aims to disrupt this power balance, and open up a wide range of roles for 'the researched person' in the research process.

Let us consider who is *doing the producing* in the production of knowledge, for example designing of the research process, the data collection and analysis, the writing, and the dissemination of research results. The standpoint of the researcher will inform – and limit – what is seen, captured and recorded (Harding, 2004). The history of disability research and the production of *disability knowledge* has largely occurred without the participation of people living with disability themselves (Stone & Priestly, 1996). Since 1975, there has been a small but consistent exploration of the emancipatory principles of inclusion (Rioux & Bach, 1994; Nind & Vinha, 2014), the idea of participatory research (Barnes & Mercer, 2004; French, 1992), and approaches to *inclusive research* involving people with intellectual disability (for example, Bigby et al, 2014; Riches, O'Brien, & The CDS Inclusive Research Network, 2017; Walmsley, Strnadova & Johnson, 2017). This echoes the approaches to participation in research by other marginalised people such as Indigenous and feminist groups. The major push in recent decades to ensure 'nothing about us, without us' (Charlton, 2000), suggests that conducting research 'on' but not 'with' people with disability, is a flawed approach.

Philosophical and practical problems occur when research is done without high level input, including leadership, from those whom the research is about (Lofgren, 2011; Johnston, 2009; Dijkers, 2009). This calls into question the validity and relevance of that research. *High quality* research studies (conforming to *gold standards* of scientific design) can fail to capture the complexity of daily life as experienced by research subjects (Dijkers, 2009). This failure manifests in limited or overly-narrow research methods, as well as research questions and priorities that may not address the issues and outcomes considered most important by those living with the experiences which are being examined (Lofgren, 2011). As Kroll argues, 'if people are systematically excluded from research participation, their needs, experiences, perspectives are rendered invisible' which skews the evidence base therefore affecting evidence-based practice (Kroll, 2011, p. 67). These issues affect a significant proportion of the rehabilitation and disability literature to date (Johnston et al, 2009; Ubel et al, 2005).

In response to this context of exclusion, participatory research has fostered a range of participation opportunities and seeks to include people with disabilities 'as more than just research subjects or respondents' (Walmsley, 2001, p.188). Roles may include 'instigators of ideas, research designers, interviewers, data analysts, authors, disseminators and users' (Walmsley & Johnson, 2003, p. 10), and in all the stages of research design, management, implementation, distribution and application of findings (Nind, 2011). In this way, the notion of participation encompasses a broad array of activities or occupations for research *subjects* including, but not limited to, as respondents.

Occupying research in *The Equipping Inclusion Studies*

The Equipping Inclusion Studies research project was commissioned by an alliance of people living with disability, assistive technology practitioners, advocates and academics in the state of Victoria, Australia. The stated concerns of the alliance became the research questions and the group hoped to provide evidence to influence government policy. The research design involved seeking the views of Victorian adults with a disability about their needs for assistive technology (AT), and the outcomes of using AT. With this beginning, the research started with solid participatory credentials. Intentional research design, such as developing an online survey method accessible for a range of AT users, was important. But as the research rolled out, research subjects, initially framed as respondents, chose to occupy a range of additional roles. It took willingness from both research subjects and researchers to explore alternate occupations or participative roles. This willingness enabled people with disability to occupy the research in the ways they did, and for this to be understood as a legitimate and valuable occupation. The research roles or occupations that were taken up in this project are summarised below.

Advisor on method

Designing for human diversity meant that one approach to data collection did not fit all respondents. For example, the qualitative approach which allowed respondents to provide in-depth descriptive comment was identified as problematic by Deafblind participants and their interpreters. Conceptual language did not translate fully into Auslan [3] and the intensive tactile communication exchange required a significant reduction of the question set. Rather than exclude Deafblind participants, the researchers enabled their engagement in the occupation of research by re-designing the research process, despite being midway through data collection. Researchers were informed by expert informants from the Deafblind community, and worked with Deafblind participants to develop a data collection method that allowed participants to engage in the occupation of research without undue burden.

Critic of data collection instruments

Use of structured and standardised tools can prevent participants from giving information they feel is important. Researchers are urged to tell participants that they are open to commentary. This may be in the form of dialogue during or after use of the formal tools. If the tools are written, researchers may structurally include some critical appraisal questions such as 'what didn't we include' and 'is there anything else to be said'. Researchers must indicate to participants that such feedback will be both heard and valued. This may challenge the idea of objectively administering data collection instruments, as well as fundamentally challenge the power relations of research, particularly who defines and classifies impairment and associated experiences, the researcher or the people living with the experience. Nevertheless, this is a critically important element if research is to be an exchange. Further, opening up an occupational role for disabled people to critique and redefine the way their experience is defined and investigated has far reaching consequences as it potentially leads to formal changes in clinical and policy understanding, focus and vocabulary.

In the following example, use of a standardised tool would have resulted in inaccurate and meaningless results without this critical dialogue. A major disability bias was evident in the mainstream health-related quality of life tool used. The continued presence of disability prevented increased scores in some quality of life domains, regardless of the health intervention provided. For example, some participants, while independently mobile using powered mobility devices, had low scores on the mobility question as they did not walk independently. Respondents identified that the tool did not reflect their experience or the positive impact of AT, and as such was inherently biased against disability. As researchers, we informed participants as to the tool's purpose and importance to the health economics component of the study, whilst simultaneously acting on this critique. Feedback was provided to the tool authors, who acknowledged that independence in this instance was conflated/equated with walking, and undertook to review the tool. Having provided their critical feedback, participants agreed to spend their time completing the tool.

Data interpreter and analyst

Throughout the data collection process, respondents created opportunities to provide analysis of their own responses. This provided researchers with a reinterpretation of the data beyond the researchers' own analyses. In practical terms this meant analysis by the researchers and an expert panel, were provided back to the participants in written and verbal formats, giving participants the chance to critique and comment on the analysis which was done.

Participants were asked to anticipate the level of improvement to their lives should an identified AT solution be provided. Many participants stated they were less satisfied with their lives once this optimal solution had been explored. One reading of this data would indicate that anticipation of optimal AT resulted in a *worse* experience, however participant informants shed a different light on this finding. Participants explained that the raising of expectations meant current life was seen as less satisfying, but also that aspiration, as a human trait, was often removed from their very rationed lives, and that the opportunity to 'think big' was appreciated. Interpretations like this were offered by several respondents and were adopted by researchers in recognition of the valid role of interpreter that respondents were undertaking as part of the research.

Ethics critic

Ethics approval requires that data be made anonymous, however some participants wished to be named in their data and stories. University ethics review processes attempt to mitigate risk for respondents by protecting anonymity. This was experienced as an assumption of vulnerability by some participants. Several participants engaged in active lobbying of researchers, and through them, of the University ethics committee, to change these requirements and give them a choice to be identified or not. This then resulted in further research-focused occupational engagement by respondents as they edited and approved case studies about themselves. Some also decided to directly participate in public events, telling their own stories related to the research topic.

Co-author, disseminator of findings and knowledge translator

Several participants sought and gained roles as co-authors of reports, magazine and journal articles, and book chapters. The occupation of authorship was empowering. For some, this enabled them to deconstruct expert knowledge and thus made peer reviewed writing more accessible. Participants also undertook a range of roles in presenting research findings to the media, policy makers and politicians, in different forums such as conferences and workshops. Some participants decided to be filmed or voice recorded and presented these films to various audiences. In some cases, participants worked for change by relating their own experiences, as captured in the research, in policy- influencing meetings. Direct communication from people living with disability, including both research participants and members of the research advisory group, altered the reception given to our study findings. Discourses or themes of rationing, (i.e. 'you want people to have the gold plated wheelchair'), changed to conversations about human rights and social justice. This is because the recipients of policy and AT funding were contributing to the change agenda by being 'in the room' and in the conversation.

In this context of the diverse roles occupied by participants, academic researchers were challenged to stand aside or alongside participants and cede or share roles. This required significant additional time in conversation and co-authorship, as well as some time in mentoring the development of these skills in some participants.

How to occupy research: The perspective of a research participant

Ricky, a research participant in *The Equipping Inclusion Studies* (Layton et al, 2010), was one of those who claimed alternate roles within the research, particularly engaging in dialogue about the inclusive / participatory / emancipatory credentials of our approach. Here is her perspective on the 'how to' of occupying research:

As a disabled person I am frequently asked to participate as a research subject, and have become picky about those invitations I accept. I have found that much of the research that's being done makes unhelpful or incorrect assumptions about my life, and even research that is good is usually just done and then uselessly forgotten about. The researchers' endless requests for disabled research participants usually assumes that we have nothing to add to their research aside from answering their pre-structured questions, and that our time is valueless – or nearly so. When I ask questions about the research prior to agreeing to take part, most researchers are shocked and they often become defensive.

These are some things that I suggest that disabled research participants think about with regards to research they're asked to participate in. Your time and energy has value and you can choose whether or not to use that time and energy on a research project:

- *What is this research about?*
  Insist on understanding the whole process, not just the part of the research that's relevant to you. Understand why the researcher is exploring this question. If the explanations use words or language that is unfamiliar or overwhelming, get them to explain it in a way that makes sense to you – researchers often use a lot of jargon without realising it.

- *Who is being researched?*
  Is this researcher taking care to include the full range of people who their research purports to be about, or are they only asking people who are easy to access? What's the point of research that only represents a small portion of the population it is about? Ask the researcher how they are working to include (as appropriate) those with more severe and multiple disabilities, those with non-English speaking backgrounds, those who live in rural and remote areas, those with psychiatric and intellectual disabilities, nonverbal people, those who are bedridden and housebound, those without internet access. What accommodations are available? How will these groups find out the research is even happening?

- *Is this research worth your time and energy?*
  What will the research results be used for? Will they just be filed in a drawer or does the researcher intend to use them to influence government policy, etc.? Research subjects are not generally paid but your time and energy still has value and worth and you should only spend it in ways that you feel are worthwhile.

- *Ensure that you have access to supports during and after*
  Research can be triggering and bring up unpleasant or upsetting thoughts and memories, even when the actual questions seem fairly innocuous. You always have the right to have a support person with you when you are interacting with researchers and/or to debrief with somebody afterwards.

- *Make the researchers deconstruct their questions, and justify the asking of the questions*
  Why do they want to know these specific things about your life? How do these questions fit into the overall piece of research? What assumptions have they made? Research, especially when done by non-disabled researchers, often doesn't ask the right questions, and misses asking about things that are important to the lives of people with disabilities because researchers don't properly understand.

- *Be non-compliant!*
  It's OK and even important to tell researchers about what they've missed asking, and it's OK to insist that they listen to the parts of your story that don't fit their questions or when your answers don't fit the format of their surveys. What they do (or don't do) with these parts will tell you a lot about how good they are, too!

- *Argue to be identified if you so choose*
  As a participant, you work hard in participating in this research and that work deserves to be acknowledged. Especially for those of us with rare disabilities, it's often clear who we are just from our answers anyway. If you would like your name used in research, speak up. This may mean the researcher has to go back and ask their ethics committee, but don't feel guilty about creating more work for them – that's their job.

- *Follow up*
- *Ask for a feedback loop, to ensure you are heard, and are 'collaborators' not just a 'sample'. You can also ask to see the text of research before it is published to make sure your perspective is properly understood.*

And if you – as a person with a disability - don't want to do these things, or can't do these things, that's OK too. It's your energy and your time and you get to choose how to spend it. If all you can manage, or all you choose to do, is answer the survey that's fine too.

What does this mean for research?

Understanding research participation as occupation brings a new value to the range of roles offered to research subjects in research. A useful framework for human functioning is provided by the *International Classification of Functioning, Disability and Health* (ICF) (WHO, 2001). The ICF provides an internationally recognised set of occupations, articulated as activities and participation chapters. Research per se as an occupation is not listed in these chapters. We suggest research is an important addition, in that it recognises the knowledge production roles of people with disability. We propose that research as occupation belongs in Chapter 8 Major Life Areas, alongside education, work and employment. We also suggest that the occupation of research represents an occupational engagement which impacts upon self-efficacy, engagement and competence across a range of other activity and participation chapters as outlined in Table 1.

Table 1
ICF Activity and Participation Chapters applicable to the occupation of research, and Sub chapter most relevant to research roles and occupation

Chapter 1 Learning and Applying Knowledge Subchapter Applying knowledge d163
Chapter 7 Interpersonal interactions and relationships Subchapter Formal relationships d740
Chapter 9 Community, social and civic life Subchapter Human rights d940 Subchapter Political life and citizenship d950

The absence of 'research' and all its roles within schema such as the ICF is evidence of the invisibility of research as occupation for people with disability. This absence justifies the sometimes assertive stance required by people with disability in order to participate more fully in research.

Understanding research participation as occupation means that researchers utilising non-participative methods must re-examine the role of respondent. Re-thinking is needed about researchers' understanding of the respondent role, as well as the values with which researchers regard respondents. If all of the above research roles are recognised as occupation, they can be understood to be meaningful and contribute to identity along with health and social inclusion outcomes. Therefore, researchers should value and facilitate these roles. This added valuing places an onus on researchers to consider how access to these roles within their research is both facilitated and denied.

Table 2 draws on a set of disability inclusive research principles to identify the breadth of occupations available to people living with disability as participants in research. These roles echo those described by Ricky, Erin and Natasha above, and should be enabled within research design.

Table 2
Australian Inclusive Research Principles (DIRC 2012).

Feature of inclusive research (Extract from DIRC 2012)	Occupational roles for research 'subjects' (examples)
Research that is informed by and/or led by people with disability The need for research, and its design, must be identified and led by people with disability.	Setting the agenda for research Identifying research questions Managing / leading research projects Advising, informing researchers
Ownership The research process, its design, management, implementation and findings must be owned by people with disability and their representative organisations.	Seeking and managing research funding Designing the research project and methods Managing or undertaking tasks within the implementation of the project Advising, writing and/or disseminating findings
Inclusive and participatory The research process, and its methodologies, must ensure that people with disability, about whom and for whom the research is designed, play a central role as researchers and as research participants; and the voice of people with disability is validated as data.	Advising on / developing accessible and inclusive methods Pilot testing methods Providing information/ data Working as researcher (data collector and/or analyst) Checking data Analysing data and advising on meaning and conclusions
Co-presenting People with disability must be provided with opportunities to present research findings.	Co-writing publications Co-presenting research findings Advocating and advising on application of findings Managing or advising on dissemination and influencing activities
Materials that are accessible Information about the research process, research tools, and research reports, must be provided in ways and in formats that are accessible.	Engaging in data provision according to capability, through diversity of materials Advising on human diversity and the nature of accessible materials

A range of types of activities Adjustment must be made to the design of research to render research appropriate to the participants and accommodate a variety of approaches (i.e. research design reflects the diversity of potential research participants). Good research design must emphasise the need for a variety of approaches to ensure that a diversity of views are researched.	Directing 'what is collected' and 'what is important' as the opinions of people with disability are the starting point for research design and method Advising on alternative methods, adjustments, or accommodations to enable participation by people with diverse disabilities Advocating for reasonable accommodations Educating researchers and linking them to appropriate resources to assist with accommodations
Research that transfers through to real life Research by and with people with disability must provide tangible benefits to individuals and the constituency of people with disability, and work toward greater inclusion of people with disability in the community.	Undertaking the role of 'critical friend' to researchers in evaluating whether research is indeed valuable from a/the disability perspective Advising on priorities and application of findings
Re-defining what research is Inclusive disability research is part of the universal research endeavour, and as such must contribute to ongoing discussions about the role and form of research in general.	Influencing 'research production' i.e. philosophy, funding priorities through advocacy Challenging ethics of non-inclusive research in various forums Developing and disseminating resources and examples of inclusive research
"The right people asking the right questions and getting the right answers" Inclusive disability research must be careful to ensure that research questions are relevant and important to people with disability (determined/informed by them), and that answers are sought from the correct sources using the best inclusive methods (i.e. identify "right people").	Developing and advising on research questions Advising on recruitment of respondents Assisting with recruitment of respondents
Consent Researchers must apply processes of ethics approval that ensure that people with disability are included in the research as willing and supportive participants.	Advising on consent issues and strategies Critiquing or challenging ethics requirements where these are inappropriate (e.g. right to be identified as a respondent)

NB Detailed examples of each element are provided in Layton, N (2014) The Practice, Research, Policy Nexus in Contemporary Occupational Therapy, *Australian Occupational Therapy Journal*, 61, 49-57

If research is an occupation, we should foster equal opportunities for participation in it by people across the spectrum of human diversity. To do this, we need to use our knowledge about overcoming barriers to occupational engagement. Aspects of standard research procedures are likely to be barriers to meaningful participation in research (e.g. ethics processes, some standardised tools, timelines) and will require occupational analysis and activity redesign. Fostering occupational opportunities in research means building in capacity for flexibility and accommodations in all potential roles. At the most basic level of enhancing opportunities to occupy the role of respondent, this will require accommodations such as:

- adapting the research tasks (e.g. are there other ways of obtaining key data which are less onerous and more suited to individual variation?);
- adapting temporal demands (e.g. short but repeated bursts of data collection; flexible according to daily needs of participants)
- designing research with accommodations for maximum human variation (e.g. alternative structures and formats for surveys, interviews; use of interpreters, circle of support, proxies, member checking).

The most important way to foster opportunities for occupational engagement is becoming open to participant perspectives about what roles are meaningful for them and the accommodations they require, if any, to occupy them. This requires explicit attention throughout the life cycle of the research project, specifically, asking for participants for their perspectives, listening for these in all interactions, and addressing them once known.

Conclusions

Research as an occupation is valuable. Our experiences demonstrate that increased occupational opportunities in research support social inclusion. This evidence suggests research belongs in a range of valued ICF participation chapters and adding research to the ICF would increase the profile of research as an occupation. Framing research participation as occupation is under-theorised and under-investigated, though the closeness-of-fit between the principles of participatory research and occupational therapy has been noted (Kramer-Roy, 2015, p.1208). Given that our social world, including the design and delivery of human services, is constructed through evidence and facts about normalcy and disability, then the valuing and occupational engagement of people whose lives are being researched is arguably the ultimate social inclusion issue.

The occupation of research has diverse elements which can be undertaken by a range of non-researchers, but it can be exclusionary in approach and practice. Research philosophies and methods can act as facilitators or barriers to people with disability engaging in the occupation of research. Challenging the notion of professional experts and taking ownership of the purpose of research demands some fundamental changes in assumptions and will challenge the status quo. A fundamental change in line with theories of universal human variation (Bickenbach, 2009) is necessary to shift current research paradigms. Instead of viewing research participants as 'other', research participants should be viewed as capable fellow humans in a life of human variation. We propose that participating in research roles is an important way to engage in health promoting occupation. Inclusive research principles offer one model to achieve this.

Notes

1. Readers may note the use of terms such as 'disabled person' instead of person living with disability; 'bedridden and housebound' instead of those who are unable to move beyond their bed or house. Many in the disability community elect to reclaim or identify with terms which are not in 'politically correct' usage. Ricky, for this chapter, directed us to avoid 'weasel words' / selected the terms when representing her views
2. www.aeaa.org.au
3. Auslan is the Australian Sign Language

References

Barnes, C. & Mercer, G. (eds) (2004) *Implementing the Social Model of Disability: Theory and Research*. Leeds, UK: The Disability Press

Bickenbach, J. (2009) Disability, culture and the UN convention. *Disability & Rehabilitation*, 31, 14, 1111–1124

Bigby, C., Frawley, P. and Ramcharan, P. (2014) Conceptualizing inclusive research with people with Intellectual Disability. *Journal of Applied Research in Intellectual Disabilities*, 27, 1, 3-12

Burchardt, T., Le Grand and Piachaud, D. (1999) Social exclusion in Britain 1991—1995. *Social Policy & Administration*, 33, 227–244

Charlton, J. (2000) *Nothing About Us Without Us: Disability oppression and empowerment*. USA: University of California Press

Disability Inclusive Research Collaboration (2012) *Quality Statement- Inclusive Research Principles*, University of Sydney, [Accessed 30 January 2015 at http://www.cdds.med.usyd.edu.au/disability-inclusive-research-principles]

Dijkers, M. (2009) *When The Best Is The Enemy Of The Good: The nature of research evidence used in systematic reviews and guidelines*. NCDDR Task Force on Systematic Review and Guidelines, National Centre for Dissemination of Disability Research [Accessed 16 August 2015 at http://www.ncddr.org/kt/products/tfpapers/tfpapers2.html]

French, S. (1992) Researching disability: The way forward. *Disability & Rehabilitation*, 14, 4, 183-186

Harding, S. (Ed.) (2004) *The Feminist Standpoint Theory Reader*. New York, USA: Routledge

Jones, K. J. Ben-David, S., & Hole, R. (2020) Are individuals with intellectual and developmental disabilities included in research? A review of the literature. *Research and Practice in Intellectual and Developmental Disabilities*, 7, 2, 99-119

Johnston, M., Vanderheiden, G., Farkas, M., Rogers, E., Summers, J.A. and Westbrook, J. (2009)

The Challenge of Evidence in Disability and Rehabilitation Research and Practice: A Position Paper. National Centre for Dissemination of Disability Research [Accessed 16 August 2015 at http://www.ncddr.org/kt/products/tfpapers/tfpapers2.html]

Kramer-Roy, D. (2015) Using participatory and creative methods to facilitate emancipatory research with people facing multiple disadvantage: A role for health and care professionals, *Disability & Society*, 30, 8, 1207-1224

Kroll, T. (2011) Designing mixed methods studies in health-related research with people with disabilities. *International Journal of Multiple Research Approaches*, 5, 1, 64-75

Layton, N., Wilson, E., Colgan, S., Moodie, M. and Carter, R. (2010) *The Equipping Inclusion Studies: Assistive technology use and outcomes in Victoria.* Melbourne, Australia: Deakin University

Law, M., Steinwender, S. and Leclair, L. (1998) Occupation, health and well-being. *Canadian Journal of Occupational Therapy*, 65, 2, 81-91

Löfgren, H., de Leeuw, E. and Leahy, M. (eds) (2011) *Democratizing Health: Consumer groups in the policy process.* Melbourne, Australia: Deakin University

Nind, M. (2011) Participatory data analysis: A step too far? *Qualitative Research*, 11, 4, 349-363

Nind, M., & Vinha, H. (2014) Doing research inclusively: Bridges to multiple possibilities in inclusive research. *British Journal of Learning Disabilities*, 42, 12, 102–109

Persson, D., Erlandsson, L.-K., Eklund, M. and Iwarsson, S. (2001) Value dimensions, meaning, and complexity in human occupation - a tentative structure for analysis. *Scandinavian Journal of Occupational Therapy*, 8, 1, 7-18

Rebeiro, K. L. (2001) Enabling occupation: The importance of an affirming environment. *Canadian Journal of Occupational Therapy*, 68, 2, 80-89

Riches, T., O'Brien, P., & The CDS Inclusive Research Network (2017). Togetherness, teamwork and challenges: "Reflections on building an inclusive research network". *British Journal of Learning Disabilities*, 45, 4, 274–281. https://doi.org/10.1111/bld.12199

Rioux, M. and Bach, M. (eds) (1994) *Disability Is Not Measles - New Research Paradigms In Disability.* New York, USA: L'Institut Roeher Institute

Stone, E. and Priestly, M. (1996) Parasites, pawns and partners: Disability research and the role of non-disabled researchers. *The British Journal of Sociology*, 47, 4, 699-716

Trentham, B., and Cockburn, L. (2005) Participatory action research. Creating new knowledge and opportunities for occupational engagement. in F.Kronenberg, S. Simo Algado and N. Pollard (Eds) *Occupational Therapy without Borders. Learning from the spirit of survivors.* Edinburgh: Elsevier (pp. 440–453)

Ubel, P., Loewenstein, G., Schwarz, N. and Smith, D. (2005) Misimagining the unimaginable: The disability paradox and health care decision making. *Health Psychology*, 24, 4, S57-S62

Unruh, A.M. (2004) Reflections on: 'so… what do you do?' Occupation and the construction of identity. *Canadian Journal of Occupational Therapy*, 71, 5, 290-295

Walmsley, J. (2001) Normalisation, emancipatory research and inclusive research in learning disability. *Disability and Society*, 16, 2,187-205

Walmsley, J. and Johnson, K. (2003) *Inclusive Research with People with Learning Disabilities: Past, present and future.* London: Jessica Kingsley

Walmsley, J., Strnadova, I., & Johnson, K.(2017) The added value of inclusive research. *Journal of Applied Research in Intellectual Disabilities*, 31, 5, 751-759. https://doi.org/10.1111/jar.12431

Whiteford, G. (2011) From occupational deprivation to social inclusion: Retrospective insights. *British Journal of Occupational Therapy*, 74, 12, 545

World Bank (2013) *Inclusion Matters: The foundation for shared prosperity.* Washington DC, USA: World Bank

World Health Organisation (2001) *International Classification of Functioning, Disability and Health.* Geneva: World Health Organisation

Wilcock, A.A. (1998) *An Occupational Perspective of Health.* New Jersey, USA: Slack

Chapter 12
Citizens participation in research: enabling citizen-researchers' collaboration

Barbara Piškur, Maarten de Wit, Barbara Casparie, Esther Stoffers, Albine Moser

Introduction

Developing participatory action research, which is based on the experience and viewpoints of citizens themselves as research partners, is rather new not only in the field of occupational therapy, but in health and social-care research in general. This chapter is about enabling citizen participation in research, (the term 'citizen' in this chapter refers to children, young people, adults, and elderly people, with and without a disability, that participate in research). The first section outlines the meanings and conceptualization of citizen participation, and the complex terminology used in the literature. The second section introduces two different conceptual models, one hierarchical model developed by Arnstein in the late sixties, and a more recent model developed by Shier, who transformed this hierarchical structure into a non-normative, dynamic model that connects levels of participation. The third section looks at the benefits, conditions and social inclusion of citizen participation in research projects, followed by the fourth section giving an example of citizen involvement and engagement in a large scale research project. The last section presents a few tools to empower citizens' collaboration in research.

Meanings and conceptualization of citizen participation in health-social care research

Professionals in education and health and social services have taken initiatives to actively involve *citizens* with and without a disability as participants in their service development and provision. The literature (Telford & Faulkner, 2004; Shea et al, 2005; Abma & Broerse, 2010; Boivin et al, 2010; Kaltoft et al, 2014; Shippee et al, 2015) also shows a growing interest in increasing citizen participation (involvement or engagement) in health and social care research.

Meanings and conceptualization of citizen participation

Participation, introduced in health - social care in 1960, has evolved as a concept through the decades with different dimensions (ILO, 2000; Nelson & Wright, 1995):

- as an end (transformational or as a process);

- as a means (instrumental or as an approach to develop).

Participation as an end (*transformational participation*) is based on the assumption that every target group bears the primary responsibility for its own development. The focus is on improving the ability of the people to participate rather than just in achieving the predetermined objectives of the project. For example, to achieve independence in daily occupations, as most often used in health care service delivery.

As a process, transformational participation is often associated with changing oppressive structures and the empowerment of citizens; it consists of various dynamic social processes, and is therefore subject to change over time. Participation is no longer seen exclusively as something in which only the target groups engage but involvement or engagement of the other stakeholders (or partners) is also important; this is also referred to as a stakeholder approach.

As a means, participation (*instrumental participation*) implies teamwork; people cooperating with each other to achieve certain goals of a (research) project more efficiently, effectively or cheaply. For example, participation through a cooperative participatory action research project can be a means of improving both a research process and research outcomes; both improvements in process and outcomes will fit target group needs.

Participation should be seen not only as a methodological instrument for technical cooperation, but also as an approach to development. This includes activities where communities are actively involved in the analysis and development of action plans for sustainable development (Cornwall, 2008).

Citizen participation in participatory action research practice means employing measures to: identify relevant citizens, share information with them, listen to their views, see them as partners, involve them in processes of development planning and decision-making, contribute to their capacity-building and, ultimately, empower them to initiate, manage and control their own self-development as well providing enabling policy for citizen participation. However, literature does not show a clear consensus on the definition of citizen participation[1]; one could say that citizen participation is organized in a diversity of ways. Arnstein (1969, p.216) wrote: 'The idea of citizen participation is a little like eating spinach: no one is against it in principle because it is good for you.'

In this chapter citizen participation for social inclusion is seen as a continuum where citizens fulfill different roles; focusing on information sharing, consultation, joint assessment, shared decision-making, collaborative mechanisms and empowering mechanisms. Social inclusion in general refers to the involvement or engagement of a wide range of citizens (including those who may easily be excluded because of their vulnerabilities) in different spheres of life by improving the accessibility to public and private services (Levitas et al, 2007). In contrast, when citizen participation lacks social integration in societal activities or occupations (e.g. research activities) as well as lacking power, this leads to social exclusion (Room, 1995) or occupational deprivation (Whiteford and Hocking, 2012).

Models of participation

Literature shows a large variety of conceptual models that can be used to portray types of citizen participation. In this chapter, two influential models are briefly presented; Arnstein's participation ladder and Shier's model of participation. Arnstein's participation ladder is hierarchical and therefore less appropriate in current application to practice that aims for social inclusion. However, several authors have been inspired by the participation ladder and developed alternative models - Shier's model is one example.

Arnstein's participation ladder

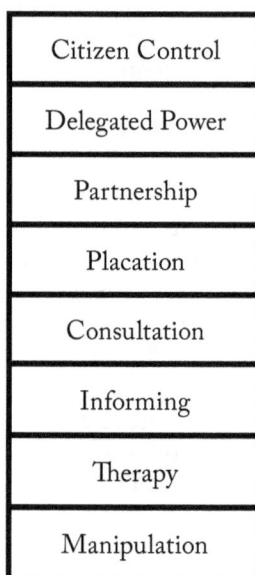

| Citizen Control |
| Delegated Power |
| Partnership |
| Placation |
| Consultation |
| Informing |
| Therapy |
| Manipulation |

Figure 1
Ladder of citizen participation (based on Arnstein, 1969).

Arnstein (1969) published the participation ladder to distinguish degrees of citizen control over decisions and to categorise different sorts of participation. The participation ladder has eight rungs, starting with the lowest ranks of non-participation (Manipulation and Therapy). A first step towards enhanced participation is tokenism (Informing, Consultation and Placation); for example, the collection of citizens' views (e.g. through surveys, interviews) and inviting citizens in advisory bodies without giving them any decision making power. Often, tokenism is referred to as paying lip-service. True citizen decision-making power is achieved in the highest three rungs (Partnership, Delegated Power and Citizen Control) of the participation ladder.

The participation ladder is widely used in different fields such as health policy (Verspaandonk, 2001) and research, like The National Advisory Group on public involvement in health research of the United Kingdom's National Institute for Health Research (NIHR).

Shier's model of participation

Shier provides a promising model (2001b) to create a 'pathway to participation' and adapts the ladder to help researchers and other stakeholders to explore the participation process, determine their current position and identify the next steps to be taken to increase their level of participation. Harry Shier's work embeds a child's right to participate in decision making into a model for involving children in participation initiatives. Shier's model (Figure 2) attempts to capture how, at each level, there may be different degrees of commitment to participation. Each level is divided into three different stages—openings, opportunities and obligations, as described by (Shier, 2001b):

- *an opening* occurs as soon as staff members make a personal statement or commitment of intent to work in a certain way. In this stage, as it is only opening, the opportunity to make it happen may not be available;
- *an opportunity*, occurs when the needs are met that will enable the staff or organization to operate at this level in practice. These needs may include resources (e.g. staff time, transport, money), skills and knowledge development of new approaches to establish tasks (e.g. available training for staff);
- *an obligation*, is established when it becomes the agreed policy of the organization or research setting that staff should operate at this level. It becomes an obligation on the staff that they must do so; it is built into the system.

The model provides a simple question for each stage of each level. In reality, it is unlikely that staff (researcher) or an organization will be tidily positioned at a single point on the diagram; they may be at different stages at different levels or at different positions in respect of different tasks.

Although this model is based on populations of children, we believe it can be applied with other 'vulnerable' populations and their organizations.

Figure 2 describes pathways to children's participation based on Shier's model of participation (2001a)

Both above mentioned conceptual models show several possibilities of citizens' participation in a research process. The first, the Arnstein ladder, takes a top-down approach in which citizens are encouraged to strive for the highest level of involvement or engagement that is meaningful to them. However, we have learned that a higher level does not necessarily mean more meaningful participation for everyone. For instance, people want to have more influence for an issue that is highly important than for an issue that is not really a priority. Also, not everyone has the same competences to act on the highest level of the ladder, some people therefore prefer the role of advisor or respondent over the role as equal partner. People want to have the freedom to choose the level of involvement that is relevant and feasible for them. The original Arnstein ladder does not take these contextual factors into account and does not allow for other ways in which citizens may want to participate.

However, it provides a clear call to citizens and researchers to avoid forms of tokenism ('pseudo-participation') and to combat unequal power relationships.

Shier's model stimulates an open dialogue about the feasibility and desirability of involvement or engagement of citizens in research by introducing three important stages (openings, opportunities and obligations). All participants are invited to discuss and agree on the level of participation in the research project, including the decision-making process.

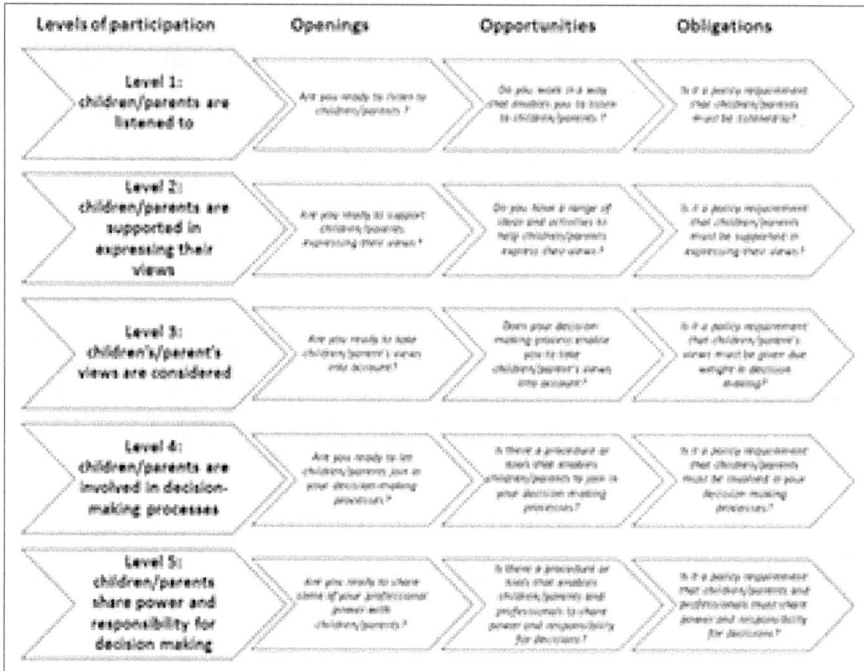

Fig 2.
Pathways to children's participation based on Shier's model of participation (2001a)

Currently in research, the most common form of citizen participation, using Arnstein's terminology, comes at the consultation/advice level, where citizens contribute to research by reading study protocols or helping to develop participant information materials. Citizens can also be involved at a collaborative level as part of the research process, helping to identify research questions and design projects. Finally, and more rarely, citizens themselves can lead research as a Chief Investigator, being the lead applicant on a grant proposal. Section 4 gives a more detailed example of citizen participation in a research project.

In education, just as in occupational therapy, Shier's model could be used as discussion tool to think about how current citizen participation in education is organized based on the three stages of the model (opening, opportunity or obligation) and what kind of conditions are needed to improve or to identify the optimum opportunity for each citizen participant.

An example of citizen participation in occupational therapy curricula:

- *an opening* - In this stage, a university occupational therapy department provides the opportunity for engagement. Staff or students are encouraged to find citizens to participate in educational activities (e.g. debate, storytelling, sharing their experience-based knowledge, being involved in examinations);
- *an opportunity*, in this stage, the occupational therapy department provide resources (e.g. staff time, transport, money), skills and knowledge development of new approaches to establish tasks for citizen participation in educational activities (e.g. available training for staff and for citizens);
- *an obligation*, this stage is established when it becomes the agreed policy of the occupational therapy department or the entire university that staff should operate at this level. It becomes an obligation for the occupational therapy staff to do educational activities together with citizens.

Benefits, conditions and policy principles of participatory health and social-care research

Benefits

Citizen participation (involvement or engagement) in research can be at every step of the research process - preparation, execution and translational phase - (Shippee et al, 2015). Participatory action research or socially inclusive research supports the possibility, the significance, and the usefulness of involving citizens in the knowledge-production process

Conditions for successful citizen participation

A core component of successful citizen participation is the building of reciprocal relationships between researchers and citizens (Young, 2014). Citizens should be involved from the very beginning as equal partners and as reliable members of the research team rather than simply as an additional variable (Shippee et al, 2015). Partnerships between researchers and citizens should include mutual understanding (Bergold & Thomas, 2012); it shows benefits for the research project, for citizens participating in research, and for the entire population:

- Ennis and Wykes (2013) found that *research projects* which involved citizens were more likely to have achieved their recruitment targets. Citizen participation in research supports researchers in commissioning, designing study protocols, focusing research that is relevant to citizens, as well choosing relevant outcomes for citizens (Beresford & Croft, 2012; Ennis & Wykes, 2013; Domecq et al, 2014). Information sheets about a research are easier to understand for potential research participants, data collection procedures are more feasible and recommendations on the timing of inclusion of research participants in the study and follow-up improve the quality of research (Boote et al, 2010).

- Furthermore, participation in research has benefits *for the citizens participating in research*, by increasing social inclusion and promoting wellbeing (NIHR; Thornicroft & Tansella, 2005), supporting empowerment and the achievement of change in line with citizens' rights, social inclusion, self-defined needs, interests, confidence, contribution, effort rewarded, and friendship (Hewlett et al, 2006).
- Last but not least, the benefits can be seen *for the entire population* by making the research and outcomes relevant to citizens (Beresford & Croft, 2012; Ennis & Wykes, 2013; Domecq et al, 2014).

Reciprocal relationships require attention to the dynamics of the learning process for all citizens and researchers, throughout the whole research process: the initial prejudices and resistance, gaining skills and getting to know each other, change in power relations and achieving mutual agreement (de Wit et al, 2015). Another condition is related to the attitude with which researchers facilitate citizen participation. A primary concern is that citizen participation in research should be genuine and not tokenistic (Domecq et al, 2014). Tokenism is lip service, which means that citizen participation is reduced to the mere fulfilment of funding requirements. As a consequence, citizens have no real impact on the research. At present, citizen participation often remains at the level of consultation (Brett et al, 2014; Wykes, 2014). A third condition for successful citizen participation in participatory action research is related to logistics, such as scheduling meetings and providing access to venues so that citizens can take part. Extra time and funding are needed for successful engagement. This should already be planned at the initiation stage. Boivin et al. (2014) found that citizen participation requires 17% more costs and 10% more time.

Research and social inclusion policy

The European Union's research policy is guided by the perceived need to gear the innovation process to societal needs and social inclusion, as suggested in the Europe 2020 strategy (Commission, 2013). Citizen participation is at the very heart of the principle of inclusiveness which directly addresses the involvement of citizens in research processes as a must and points at the responsibility of researchers (Hennen & Pfersdorf, 2014). However, research (e.g. (Jørgensen, 2011) shows variations in the extent to which research informs inclusive policy. For example in this research (Jørgensen, 2011) the role of expert knowledge in integration policy-making in the case of Sweden and Denmark has been investigated. The two countries have developed very different integration policies and therefore provide an interesting comparison of the research–policy relationship. In Sweden, social scientists have been influential in agenda-setting and conceptual rethinking of immigrant integration policies. In Denmark social science research has been utilized in a more selective pick-and-choose manner to take only what is wanted to legitimate government policies (Jørgensen, 2011). Therefore, it is important to mention that in order to provide full-bodied evidence to support socially inclusive practice, research methods themselves must be socially inclusive. For example, research that excludes certain population groups from research participation due to language barriers does not support full social inclusion of all citizens.

Example of a research project portraying citizen participation

This section provides a practical example of citizen participation (involvement and / or engagement) in a research project. The intensity of citizen participation has been described according to the terminology of the participation ladder of Arnstein. The dynamic of the process of citizen participation has been described as portrayed in Shier's model.

Parents' role in enabling the participation of children with a physical disability

Parents' role in enabling the participation of children with a physical disability (Piškur, 2015) is an example of a PhD project that took the tenet *'Nothing about us without us'* as a guiding principle. In 2010, very little information was available in the Netherlands on how to support the process of citizen involvement or engagement in research, or how to support researchers in this process.

Citizen participation in this research project took place in several meaningful ways:

- a mother of a child with a Cerebral palsy (BC), as a co-researcher (shared power and responsibility for decision-making);
- a parent organization – BOSK - (involved in decision-making processes);
- a parents' panel (views taken into account and supported in expressing their views);
- study participants in three empirical studies (were listened to).

How have these ways been achieved? First, the primary investigator (BP), who previously worked together with a mother of a child with a CP (BC) in a post graduate occupational therapy education, explored the innovative idea of citizen involvement in research with her. Together, the primary investigator, the mother (BC), researchers and representatives of the parent organisation (BOSK) formulated the main theme of the entire project. The mother (BC) was also a member of a parent organisation and encouraged that a larger parent panel should be involved in different stages of the project. This also led to the involvement of the entire parent organisation. Each of them took a different role and meaning in the project. Table 1 shows a matrix with examples from three research projects (Piškur, 2015), describing vertically the five possible roles of citizen participation in research, as described in the participation model of Shier (2001b) and horizontally the different stages of the research cycle.

Several steps followed before the mother (BC) became a co-researcher. First, she completed a job application procedure and took part in a job interview. To learn more about her role as a co-researcher, she followed the training programme organised by TOOLS2use, a patient led association to support and educate patient research partners (TOOLS). This training programme empowered her to recognize and fulfil her role as a citizen in a large scale research project at first place and not as a researcher. She often expressed: *'I am not a researcher, but I know very well how this feels for parents, like me'*. Some examples follow for each level of the participation ladder.

Table 1
Matrix from three research projects

Level of involvement	Preparation phase			Execution phase		Translation phase		
	Agenda setting	Study design & procedures	Study recruitment	Data collection	Data analysis	Dissemination	Implementation	Evaluation
Shared power and responsibility for decision-making		A* B* C*			B* C*	A* B* C*	A* B* C*	A* B* C*
Involved in decision-making processes	A* B* C*		A* B* C*	A* B* C*	A*			
Views taken into account			A^ B^ C^			A^ B* C^	A^B^ C^	
Supported in expressing their views		A^ B^ A" B"						
Listen to				A# B# C#	C#			

Legend: A – survey study, B – diary study, C – phenomenological study, * = Mrs. B. Casparie, = BOSK, " = parents' panel, # = study participant

Shared power and responsibility for decision-making

In the design of the survey study (Piškur et al, 2015), the mother (BC) was in control of decision-making. Several discussions took place about instruments that could be included in the parent questionnaire. She was able to think both from a perspective of the larger community (other parents of children with a disability) she represented and also from her role in research, as expressed in the following quote:

> *'I know you suggested to use a particular valid instrument as a part of the parent questionnaire, but some questions in this instrument were rather negative, almost aggressive...this is not very nice for parents...for me personally something like this makes me decide to throw it in the bin.'*

Based on her advice, the team included a different instrument in the questionnaire.

Another example that illustrates her role of sharing power and responsibility was the analysis process in the phenomenological study. During the process of describing the findings, she challenged the research team about their naming of the themes. In her opinion, the names given to the themes did not fully capture the experiences of the parents; they were understated. Based on her remarks and suggestions the names of the themes were changed. This small example illustrates an ongoing process of discussion between the mother and the research team until the entire group reached consensus. Finally, BC chose the appropriate names for the major themes portraying the results of the study.

Involved in decision-making processes

Agenda setting and the conceptualisation of the project stages were done in collaboration. At first this research project aimed to collect a large amount of quantitative data; the mother was sceptical 'if we could learn enough from collecting numbers'. In her opinion numbers and statistics is one way of portraying needs of parents, but it is more important to be able to describe their underlying concerns. She suggested the project also use a qualitative approach in which we could ask parents about their needs, concerns or successful strategies to enable participation that worked for their children. The design was changed to a mixed method inquiry, using a sequential data collection approach with an extensive qualitative part. One example was the design of the folder for parents. BC stressed that for study participants it is important 'to become motivated for a study and think that they personally can contribute to it' and therefore information that encourages participation should come first in a folder. The survey design and the sequence of the questions in the parent questionnaire are other examples that were influenced by BC's involvement; she was convinced that a good structure would be to have the 'first questions should be related to the aim of the study and at the end provide the demographic information'. She explained to us that most of the surveys she received at that time promised to focus on a particular research topic but she would have to answer one to two pages of demographic information before knowing what it was about. In her opinion, this did not encourage research participants; the research focus should be first, additional information should come at the end.

Citizen views taken into account and supported in expressing their views

The parent organisation also took part in this research project. Their role was to advise on different stages of the research process. For example, the average response rate of parents who have children with a physical disability is often low because they have limited opportunities to participate in studies. The parent organisation gave very good advice for a successful recruitment strategy and dissemination of results by promoting the study during a parent congress. This resulted in a follow-up national parent project called in Dutch 'Schouders' (meaning 'shoulders') that includes not only motivated and active parents, but also those who are usually not involved.

Citizen are supported in expressing their views

The parent panel consisted of 12 members. They were consulted in the preparation phases of different studies to provide us with feedback on the study design and expressed their views about study materials.

Citizens are listened to

The mother (BC), the parent panel and the study participants shared their views on the different studies and helped to distribute information through social media (e.g. Facebook and blogs).

The four-year journey with the parents in this thesis project has been significant in many ways. The research team learned:

- to be able to work together as a team and to take mutual decisions (needing open dialogue, equal positions and critical reflection);
- how to involve the citizen as co-researcher in all stages of the research process to improve its quality (e.g. by realising that not every validated assessment instrument is user friendly);
- to understand each other's language and to appreciate each unique contribution to the research process (research language is not always easy to follow for a citizen);
- about the amount of effort and organisation user involvement may take (e.g. some meetings were held in Eindhoven - one-and-a-half-hour drive with a car - and due to practical reasons the mother was not able to join all those meetings).

Also for the co-researcher (the mother - BC) this journey has been noteworthy in many ways:

- in the research project, she initiated several dissemination actions, such as suggesting where to publish study results that other parents of children with a disability could access;
- in her personal life, she got new insights from the study results and used them in her daily life (e.g. tried out actions that parents in different studies described to enable their child's participation in daily life);
- she took a new role as representative on a client-board in a rehabilitation centre to be able to support other parents or clients in similar situations.

Active citizen involvement in research also showed some issues to be considered in future research projects:

- financial aspects, such as payment in order to feel equal; she is not an employee of the research centre but an external contributor of a research centre. Most citizens involved in research have some sort of social security benefits; when they accept an additional job they risk losing those benefits;
- the necessity to have a policy or a white paper about citizen involvement or engagement in research.

Tools to empower citizens and researchers to collaborate

Structural citizen participation in research requires the long term commitment between citizens and researchers as well as consistent integration of experience-based knowledge in each phase of the research project (de Wit, 2013; INVOLVE). Therefore, tools to support citizens in research and researchers themselves are needed. The following sections provide the reader with some examples of practical tools that have been developed over the last years for citizens and researchers, followed by conditions for citizen participation.

Enabling citizens to collaborate

The traditional forms of research carried out by dominant groups can be oppressive both in terms of their processes or/and outcomes; those research studies have done too little to improve lives of the citizens (Oliver, 1992; Barnes, 2003; Frankham, 2009). In contrast to these approaches, the emancipatory disability research agenda warrants the generation and production of meaningful and accessible knowledge about the various structures – economic, political, cultural and environmental – that create and sustain the multiple deprivations encountered by the majority of citizens (Frankham, 2009). Participatory Action Research (PAR) is an approach to research which empowers citizens and the community to define their own research questions, lead the process of investigation, and create their own solutions for change. Through this process, citizens and the community build skills and capacity, are able to participate in decisions affecting their lives, and engage in interactions and relationship building – all of which are the defining conditions of social inclusion. From this perspective the role of the researcher is to help facilitate these goals through the research process; for example, by using communication aids to create opportunities for citizens or children who are communicatively vulnerable (e.g. pictograms or adapted informed consent forms). Another example is photo-voice, a participatory action research approach that enables research involvement of people with low literacy skills. Several methods (e.g. nominal group discussion) and tools (e.g. participatory mapping tool – more information will be provided in the next paragraph) to support PAR, especially when little is known about the research area, have been developed; these are currently used in the field of education and development of interventions (Kathirvel et al, 2012).

Participatory tools

Participatory social mapping is an interactive approach that draws on local people's knowledge, enabling citizens to create visual and non-visual data to explore social problems, opportunities and research questions (Bergold & Thomas, 2012). Citizens work together to create a visual representation of a place using the tools and materials at their disposal. At the same time, while creating their map, the group may deliberate over how to best represent the place in the research question, share their observations as they go along, and tell personal stories and anecdotes. This can lead to rich and sometimes surprising data for health and social care research. At the same time it actively involves citizens in the process of setting the research agenda.

Especially, very vulnerable groups, like children need to be facilitated by using participatory methods and creating conditions to enable their participation in research. An example would be *Body mapping* (likes and dislikes), which could be applied as an icebreaker or introductory tool to help understand children's likes and dislikes about a topic or situation (O'Kane, 2013). A simple monitoring and evaluation tool '*H' Assessment* would be appropriate when exploring the strengths (or successes) and weaknesses (or challenges) of any initiative/ group / process and to suggest action ideas to improve the same (Giertsen, 2008).

Enabling researchers for citizen involvement

In 2013, in cooperation with Dr. Maarten de Wit (service-user and expert in service-user involvement) and 'Huis voor de Zorg', Zuyd University, The Netherlands, started a new initiative called *'Enabling researchers for citizen involvement'*. This initiative to promote citizen involvement in research, comprised the following steps: a master class for researchers, educators, citizens and students, to set the scene, which was guided by a participatory expert; followed by an independent assignment for the researchers that signed in for the 'Enabling researchers program' to briefly present their research project and the role of the citizen involvement; several coaching sessions that included (a) discussion on the important elements of citizen participation, the added value of citizen participation and individual researcher's expectations, (b) thinking about which citizens fit with the individual research project, and what are the criteria for the job application to become, for example, a co-researcher, (c) ideal citizen participation using a template for citizen involvement based on the participation ladder (de Wit et al, 2018). The template can be used as a tool to support research teams in identifying the possible roles and tasks of citizen involvement throughout the entire research process (see example in Table 1), (d) reflection on the implementation process and its related supporting and obstructing factors such as (e) discussing the sustainability of the citizen involvement in a research project and (f) evaluating in a joint session with citizens and researchers the 'Enabling researcher program' - see Figure 3. However, to enable researchers for citizen involvement a 'soft' and a 'hard' structure is needed. By 'soft' structure we mean a positive attitude and a participation culture. By a 'hard' structure we mean general agreements such as a statement of commitment, implementation of a policy concerning citizen participation in research and funding to support citizen participation while preparing a research component. The detailed results of the program will be published soon.

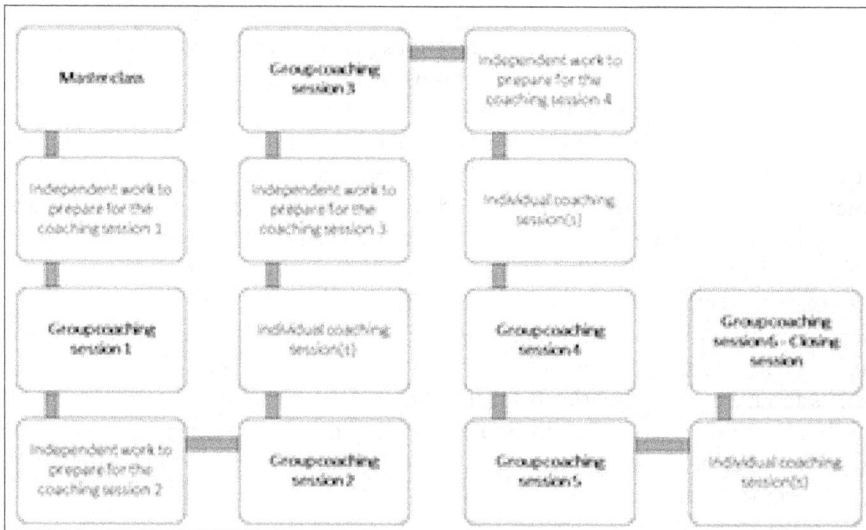

Critical appraisal guidelines for assessing the quality and impact of citizen involvement in research.

Wright et al. (Wright et al, 2010) developed a tool with nine appraisal criteria to assess quality and impact of citizen involvement in research. Criteria include issues such as '*Is the rationale for involving users clearly demonstrated?*', '*Is the level of user involvement appropriate?*', '*Is the recruitment strategy appropriate?*', and '*Is the nature of training appropriate?*' as presented in the Table 2.

When assessing the quality of user involvement in funding proposals, the purpose of the criteria is to indicate the level of skills of the research team and the quality of the proposed framework for engaging with users.

Conditions for citizen participation: training and support

Tailoring training and support for citizen involvement or engagement in research is helpful and constructive (INVOLVE, 2012). The Resource Centre of the INVOLVE describes training as different kinds of learning opportunities including group sessions with a trainer, providing high quality written materials and guidance, learning on-the-job, attending conferences, networking and shared learning with peers, online activities, university or college courses. It is important to remember that those receiving training, whether researchers or citizens, will come with a wide range of skills and experience. Support is described as a wide range of activities that enable citizens and researchers to work together: practical and financial issues, emotional and psychological support, project supervision to promote professionals, and personal development.

In our opinion, research institutes need to develop family friendly (inclusive) policies to enable citizens–researchers' collaboration. Those policies need to address aspects, such as: citizen support to balance work and family roles; costs, quality and time constraint issues at different stages of the project, and providing opportunities for those citizens to grow as research partners.

Figure 3
Enabling researchers for citizen involvement process

Research activity	Appraisal criteria	Write comments here
Planning and project design	1. Is the rationale for involving users clearly demonstrated? Consider the following: (a) Have the researchers explained the rationale for user involvement?	
	2. Is the level (e.g. partnership or consultation) of user involvement appropriate? Consider the following: (a) Have the researchers explained and justified the level of user involvement? (e.g. have they discussed whether the study involves user consultation, user collaboration or user control?) (b) Have the researchers discussed the nature of tasks users were asked to perform (e.g. identifying the research question, selecting the research method, commenting on information sheets, data collection, data analysis, dissemination?)	
Recruitment and training	3. Is the recruitment strategy appropriate? Consider the following: (a) Have the researchers explained how users have been identified? (b) Have attempts been made to involve a wide cross-section of interests where appropriate (e.g. ethnic minorities, age, gender)? (c) Have the researchers discussed the credentials of the users involved? (E.g. Do the researchers discuss why the users involved are appropriate to meeting the aims of the involvement activity?)	
	4. Is the nature of training appropriate? Consider the following: (a) Have the researchers discussed the nature of the training provided? (b) Is the nature and extent of the training justified by the researchers? (e.g. Do the researchers discuss how the training meets the needs of the users during the course of the study?) (c) Has an account been given of user involvement training for professional researchers, where necessary?	
Data collection and analysis	5. Has sufficient attention been given to the ethical considerations of user involvement and how these were managed? Consider the following: (a) Do the researchers discuss ethical issues relating to the involvement of users in research? (e.g. fatigue, the emotional demands of data collection)? (b) Are there any discussions about the management of ethical issues (e.g. provision of adequate information about research tasks, peer supervision)?	
	6. Has sufficient attention been given to the methodological considerations of user involvement and how these were managed? Consider the following: (a) Have the researchers discussed methodological issues relating to user involvement in research (e.g. potential impact on the quality of the data)? (b) Do the researchers discuss how methodological issues are managed (e.g. how differences in interpretation of qualitative data are negotiated?)	
Dissemination	7. Have there been any attempts to involve users in the dissemination of findings? Consider the following: (a) Have users been involved in the writing of the publication / funding application? (b) Have the researchers described how the findings have been disseminated to participants and service users? (c) Are findings disseminated appropriately where necessary (e.g. translation of findings into different languages, provision of interim findings to participants in receipt of palliative care)?	
Evaluation and impact assessment	8. Has the added-value of user involvement been clearly demonstrated? Consider the following: (a) Do the researchers discuss what difference involving users in the design and conduct of the research has made to the research process? (i.e. Have the researchers considered whether the study and findings would look any different if users were not involved)? (b) Do the researchers support the claims for the benefits of user involvement with examples from the research project?	
	9. Have there been any attempts to evaluate the user involvement component of the research? Consider the following: (a) Have the researchers discussed the evaluation of the impact of user involvement on the research project (e.g. impact on the design of the study, the financial cost of involvement activities, cost-benefit analyses)? (b) Do the researchers support claims about the impact of user involvement with examples from the evaluation?	

Concluding remarks

Citizen participation in research is a process that needs to be meaningful, custom made, and allowing different forms or levels of participation. Readiness for mutual learning and a structural approach promote sustainable relationships between citizens and researchers; it requires an extra effort in terms of time, money and energy in which the role of the project leader is crucial. Occupational therapists, by their own espousal of client centred practice, should be able to embrace the notion of citizen participation in occupational therapy research, as well as in education and practice. Moreover, the times are changing; occupational therapy will have to consider that citizen participation is fundamental and that 'Nothing About Us Without Us' is a must for meeting the needs of citizens (Piškur, 2013), also in research.

Note

1   Webster's definition of participation (Merriam-Webster Dictionary, 201.) describe it as the means to have a share in common with others, to partake with others; direct citizen participation would alternatively mean fulfillment of one's legal rights and duties as specified in the constitution, or alternatively, active involvement in substantive issues of government and community (Boivin, A., Currie, K., Fervers, B., Gracia, J., James, M., Marshall, C., Sakala, C., Sanger, S., Strid, J., Thomas, V., Van Der Weijden, T., Grol, R. & Burgers, J. 2010. Patient and public involvement in clinical guidelines: international experiences and future perspectives. Quality and Safety in Health Care, 19, e22.. Sherry Arnstein's ARNSTEIN, S. R. 1969. A ladder of citizen participation. Journal of the American Institute of Planners, 35, 216-224.) definition of participation incorporates substantive interests of the society, such as race, class, and gender, to define citizen participation as a categorical term for citizen power.

References

Abma, T. A. and Broerse, J. E. W. (2010) Patient participation as dialogue: Setting research agendas. *Health Expectations*, 13, 160-173

Arnstein, S. R. (1969) A ladder of citizen participation. *Journal of the American Institute of Planners*, 35, 216-224

Barnes, C. (2003) What a difference a decade makes: Reflections on doing 'emancipatory' disability research. *Disability and Society*, 18, 3-17

Beresford, P. and Croft, S. (2012) *User Controlled Research: Scoping review.* London: NHR

Bergold, J. and Thomas, S. (2012) *Participatory Research Methods: A methodological approach in motion.* 2012, 13

Boivin, A., Currie, K., Fervers, B., Gracia, J., James, M., Marshall, C., Sakala, C., Sanger, S., Strid, J., Thomas, V., Van Der Weijden, T., Grol, R. and Burgers, J. (2010) Patient and public involvement in clinical guidelines: international experiences and future perspectives. *Quality and Safety in Health Care*, 19, e22

Boivin, A., Lehoux, P., Lacombe, R., Burgers, J. & Grol, R. (2014) Involving patients in setting priorities for healthcare improvement: A cluster randomized trial. *Implementation Science,* **9,** 1-10

Boote, J., Baird, W. and Beecroft, C. (2010) Public involvement at the design stage of primary health research: a narrative review of case examples. *Health Policy,* **95,** 10 - 23

Brett, J., Staniszewska, S., Mockford, C., Herron-Marx, S., Hughes, J., Tysall, C. and Suleman, R. (2014) Mapping the impact of patient and public involvement on health and social care research: a systematic review. *Health Expectations,* **17,** 637-650

Cornwall, A. (2008) Unpacking 'participation': Models, meanings and practices. *Community Development Journal,* **43,** 269-283

De Wit, M. (2013) *Patient participation in rheumatology research: A four level responsive evaluation.* PhD, Vrije Universiteit.

de Wit, M., Beurskens, A., Piškur, B., Stoffers, E., & Moser, A. (2018) Preparing researchers for patient and public involvement in scientific research: Development of a hands-on learning approach through action research. *Health Expect,* **21,** 4, 752-763. doi:10.1111/hex.12671

De Wit, M. P. T., Elberse, J. E., Broerse, J. E. W. and Abma, T. A. (2015) Do not forget the professional – the value of the FIRST model for guiding the structural involvement of patients in rheumatology research. *Health Expectations,* **18,** 489-503

Domecq, J., Prutsky, G., Elraiyah, T., Wang, Z., Nabhan, M., Shippee, N., Brito, J., Boehmer, K., Hasan, R., Firwana, B., Erwin, P., Eton, D., Sloan, J., Montori, V., Asi, N., Abu Dabrh, A. M. and Murad, M. (2014) Patient engagement in research: a systematic review. *BMC Health Services Research,* **14,** 89

Ennis, L. & Wykes, T. (2013) Impact of patient involvement in mental health research: longitudinal study. *The British Journal of Psychiatry,* **203,** 381-386

European Commission (2013) *Guide To Social Innovation.* Brussels: Regional and Urban Policy, European Commission

Frankham, J. (2009) *Partnership Research: A review of approaches and challenges in conducting research in partnership with service users.* Manchester: Manchester Metropolitan University

Giertsen, A. (2008) *A Kit of Tools: For participatory research and evaluation with children.* Norway: Save the Children

Hennen, L. and Pfersdorf, S. (2014) Public Engagement - Promises, demands and fields of practice. *Engaging Society in Horizon 2020.* Engage2020-2014

Hewlett, S., Wit, M., Richards, P., Quest, E., Hughes, R., Heiberg, T. and Kirwan, J. (2006) Patients and professionals as research partners: Challenges, practicalities, and benefits. Arthritis and Rheumatism, 55, 676-680

International Labour Organisation (ILO) (2000) Key Concepts in Participatory Approaches. Geneva: International Labour Organisation

INVOLVE. (n.d.) Website Support Public Involvement in NHS, Public Health and Social Care Research. National Institute for Health Research. [Accessed 20 September 2015 at http://involve.co.uk/services/involvement-tools-programmes/].

INVOLVE (2012) Developing Training and Support for Public Involvement in Research. Eastleigh: INVOLVE.

Jørgensen, M. B. (2011) Understanding the research–policy nexus in Denmark and Sweden: The field of migration and integration. The British Journal of Politics & International Relations, 13,1, 93-109

Kaltoft, M., Nielsen, J., Salkeld, G. and Dowie, J. (2014) Increasing user involvement in health care and health research simultaneously: A proto-protocol for 'person-as-researcher' and online decision support tools. JMIR Research Protocols, 3, e61

Kathirvel, S., Jeyashree, K. and Patro, B. K. (2012) Social mapping: A potential teaching tool in public health. Medical Teacher, 34, e529-e531

Levitas, R., Pantazis, C., Fahmy, E., Gordon, D., Lloyd, E. and Patsios, D. (2007) The Multi-Dimensional Analysis Of Social Exclusion. Bristol, UK: Bristol Institute for Public Affairs, University of Bristol

Merriam Webster Disctionary (2015) Participate.

Nelson, N. & Wright, S. (1995) Power and Participatory Development: Theory and Practice, London, Intermediate Technology Publications: Amazon Giveaway

NIHR National Institute for Health Research (INVOLVE project). http://www.invo.org.uk/

Oliver, M. (1992) Changing the social relations of research production. Disability, Handicap and Society, 7, 101-115

O'Kane, C. (2013) Children's Participation in the Analysis, Planning and Design of Programmes: A guide for Save the Children staff. London: Save the Children Fund. Accessed 22nd April 2022 at https://resourcecentre.savethechildren.net/document/childrens-participation-analysis-planning-and-design-programmes-guide-save-children-staff/

Piškur, B. (2013). Social participation: Redesign of education, research, and practice in occupational therapy. Scandinavian Journal of Occupational Therapy, 20, 2-8

Piškur, B. (2015) Parents' role in enabling the participation of their child with a physical disability: Actions, challenges and needs. PhD, Maastricht University.

Piškur, B., Beurskens, A. J. H. M., Jongmans, M. J., Ketelaar, M. and Smeets, R. J. E. M. (2015) What do parents need to enhance participation of their school-aged child with a physical disability? A cross-sectional study in the Netherlands. Child: Care, Health and Development, 41, 84-92

Room, G. (1995) Beyond the Threshold: The measurement and analysis of social exclusion. Bristol: The Policy Press

Shea, B., Santesso, N., Qualman, A., Heiberg, T., Leong, A., Judd, M., Robinson, V., Wells, G., Tugwell, P. and The Cochrane Musculoskeletal Consumer Group (2005) Consumer-driven health care: Building partnerships in research. Health Expectations, 8, 352-359

Shier, H. (2001a) Pathways to participation: openings, opportunities and obligations. Children & Society, 15, 107-117

Shier, H. (2001b) Pathways to participation: Openings, opportunities and obligations - a new model for enhancing children's participation in decision-making, in line with article 12.1 of the United Nations Convention on the Rights of the Child. Children and Society 15, 107-117

Shippee, N. D., Domecq Garces, J. P., Prutsky Lopez, G. J., Wang, Z., Elraiyah, T. A., Nabhan, M., Brito, J. P., Boehmer, K., Hasan, R., Firwana, B., Erwin, P. J., Montori, V. M. and Murad, M. H. (2015) Patient and service user engagement in research: a systematic review and synthesized framework. Health Expectations, 18, 1151-1166

Telford, R. and Faulkner, A. (2004) Learning about service user involvement in mental health research. Journal of Mental Health, 13, 549-559

Thornicroft, G. and Tansella, M. (2005) Growing recognition of the importance of service user involvement in mental health service planning and evaluation. Epidemiologia e Psichiatria Sociale, 1-3

TOOLS. (n.d.) TOOLS: Patient empowerment. Europees deskundigen netwerk. [Accessed 12 January 2010 at http://tools2use.eu/netwerkN.html]

Verspaandonk, R. (2001) *Shaping Relations between Government and Citizens: Future Directions in Public Administration*. Research paper. Canberra: Parliamentary Library.

Whiteford, G. E. and Hocking, C. (2012) *Occupational Science: Society, inclusion, participation*, West Sussex, Wiley-Blackwell

Wright, D., Foster, C., Amir, Z., Elliott, J. and Wilson, R. (2010) Critical appraisal guidelines for assessing the quality and impact of user involvement in research. *Health Expectations*, 13, 359-368

Wykes, T. (2014) Great expectations for participatory research: what have we achieved in the last ten years? *World Psychiatry*, 13, 24-27

Young, E. (2014) *Evaluation Of The Impact Of The Free Movement Of EU Citizens At Local Level*. European Commisson: Accessed 22nd April 2022 at: http://www.barkauk.org/news/evaluation-of-the-impact-of-the-free-movement-of-eu-citizens-at-local-level/

Index

Note: Page locators in *italic* refer to figures or photographs.

Buddhism 29
Burchardt, T. 135

Canada
    Aboriginal health and occupation inequities 120–121, 122
    Aboriginal population groups 121–122
    assimilationist education policy 123–124, 129, 130
    reserve communities 122, 126
    residential schools 123–124, 129
    see also First Nations youth 'Educational Vision Quests' Photovoice project
Chamberlain, P. 99, 100, 102, 104, 105
children experiencing early adversity, enhancing occupational potential and health
    for 11–25
    applying LCHD model 11–12, 13, 14, 18, 20
    delayed permanency 12–13
    early intervention programs 14–15
    family homelessness 13–15
    implications for occupational therapy 18–20, *19*
    residential segregation and racism 15–17
    toxic stress 11, 14
        and early family bonding 17–18
children with a disability, research participation for
    Parents' role in enabling the participation of children with a physical disability 157–160
    participatory tools 161
    Shier's model of participation 153, 154, *154*, 157, *158*
CIL-Kathmandu (Independent Living Centre - CIL) 66–75
    achievements 71–72
    activities 69–70
    collaborations with civil society 67
    contemporary issues 72–74
    Disability Rights campaigning 66–67, *67*, 69, *69*, 71
    government relationship with 68
    history 66–67
    international community links 68
    objectives and activities 69–70
    participation in people's movement of 2006 67, 71
    vision, mission and goals 68, *69*
client councils 108–109
    challenges of co-determination 110
    rights 109–110
    WMCZ 1996 and 108, 109, 110–111, 118
    WMCZ 2018 and 108–109, 109–110, 118
client councils, GGZinGeest research study 111–118
    analytic approach 113–114

Young Africa 59–60

Zimbabwe *see* legislative framework in Zimbabwe to promote occupation-based
  social inclusion
Zimbabwean Association of Occupational Therapists (ZAOT) 59